Nutrition and Disease Management in Poultry

Nutrition and Disease Management in Poultry

Quentin Perez
Editor

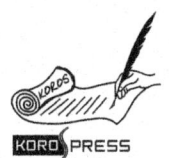

KOROS PRESS LIMITED
London, UK

Nutrition and Disease Management in Poultry

© 2012
Printed in 2017 for Sale in the Indian Subcontinent

Published by
Koros Press Limited
3 The Pines, Rubery B45 9FF, Rednal,
Birmingham, United Kingdom

Tel.: +44-7826-930152
Email: info@korospress.com
www.korospress.com

ISBN: 978-1-78163-193-5

Editor: Quentin Perez

Printed in UK

10 9 8 7 6 5 4 3 2 1

British Library Cataloguing in Publication Data
A CIP record for this book is available from the British Library

Exclusively distributed by CBS Publishers & Distributors Pvt. Ltd.
Sales & Distribution Rights only for India, Pakistan, Bangladesh, Sri Lanka, Nepal and Bhutan.This book is not to be sold outside these territories.

Contents

6. Chicken Anaemia Virus Infection 181

Chicken Infectious Anaemia, Blue Wing Disease, Anaemia Dermatitis Syndrome, Hemorrhagic Aplastic Anaemia Syndrome • Dissecting Aneurysm • Inclusion Body Hepatitis Hydropericardium Syndrome • Perirenal Hemorrhage Syndrome of Turkeys • Round Heart Disease of Turkeys • Candidiasis • Cryptosporidiosis • Coronaviral Enteritis of Turkeys

7. Duck Viral Enteritis 201

Duck Plague • Hexamitiasis • Necrotic Enteritis • Rotaviral Infections in Chickens, Turkeys, and Pheasants • Trichomoniasis • Ulcerative Enteritis • Avian Campylobacter Infection • Avian Chlamydiosis • Avian Nephritis Viral Infections

8. Avian Spirochetosis 221

Avian Borreliosis • Listeriosis • Malabsorption Syndrome • Mycoplasmosis • Mycoplasma Iowae Infection • Mycoplasma Meleagridis Infection • Mycoplasma Synoviae Infection • Salmonelloses • Pullorum Disease • Fowl Typhoid • Arizona Infection • Paratyphoid Infections • Tuberculosis • Infectious Bronchitis • Miscellaneous Conditions of Poultry • Gout • Colibacillosis • Duck Viral Hepatitis • Enterococcosis • Erysipelas

Preface

Local chickens are kept in many parts of the world irrespectively of the climate, traditions, life standard, or religious taboos relating to consumption of eggs and chicken meat like those for pig meat. To the poor majority in rural areas, local chickens serve as an immediate source of meat and income when money is needed for urgent family needs. It constitutes a significant contribution to human livelihood and contributes significantly to food security. Women and sometimes youths are the mostly involved in keeping these chickens. The local chickens are known for various merits.

Most important, they are known for their adaptation superiority in terms of their resistance to endemic diseases and other harsh environmental conditions. However, local chickens are poor performers in terms of growth rate and egg production. Most of them are of small adult size and lay small sized eggs when compared to improved commercial broiler or layer birds respectively. What is generally referred to as local chickens is a pool of heterogeneous individuals which differ in adult body size, weight and plumage. They are of several ecotypes that are distinct. Their performance vary considerably and no single ecotype meets the attributes of good egg traits, fertility, hatchability, survivability, high growth rate, heavy weight at slaughter and high egg production. Fortunately, their genetic diversity could be exploited to improve their productivity. It is therefore a laudable proposition that more attention should be given to the genetic improvement and development of the local chicken in order to ameliorate the present acute animal protein shortage to many poor societies around the globe. One way of improving the local chicken is by cross breeding with improved commercial breeds. In Nigeria, cross breeding local fowls to commercial Rhode Island Red chicken produced Fulani-ecotype chicken that is superior to other local ecotypes within Nigeria in terms of egg traits, hatchability, growth performance and live weight. Such improvements provide potentially good ecotypes for meat and egg production and could thus help to develop improved local strains. Studies on improvement of local chickens are rarely reported in other parts of the world including Tanzania. Stemming on the importance of local chicken to the economy of the poor majority in Tanzania, this study was designed to gather preliminary information on the feasibility of improving the local chicken by cross breeding with the commercial RIR. The study explored and compared egg traits, fertility, hatchability, chick hatch weight, and chick survivability for local, RIR, and crossbred chickens.

This book is prepared as a practical guide for both large and small poultry keepers and those interested in starting a poultry enterprise.

—Editor

Chapter 1

Epidemic Threat from Poultry Farming

Bird Flu is a Real Pandemic Threat to Humans

As their lungs filled ... the patients became short of breath and increasingly cyanotic. After gasping for several hours they became delirious and incontinent, and many died struggling to clear their airways of a blood-tinged froth that sometimes gushed from their nose and mouth. It was a dreadful business.

Isaac Starr, 3rd year medical student, University of Pennsylvania, 1918.

All the genes of all influenza viruses in the world are being maintained in aquatic birds, and periodically they transmit to other species... The 1918 viruses are still being maintained in the bird reservoir. So even though these viruses are very ancient, they still have the capacity to evolve, to acquire new genes, new hosts. The potential is still there for the catastrophe of 1918 to happen again.

Dr. Robert Webster, Influenza Expert, Present Day.

The pair of quotes presented above were used to begin and end a short essay I wrote many years ago on The 1918 Spanish Flu Pandemic. Isaac Starr's words offer powerful testimonial to the harsh lethality of a killer stain of influenza, and Dr. Robert Websters observation reminds us that it would be dangerous to regard the events of 1918 as an isolated slice of history that we can safely file away and forget.

In the early part of 1995, as I cast around in search of the disease that would ultimately prove to be the true villian of the science thriller I was planning to write, influenza was scarcely on the radar scope of anyone but virologists specialising in the field of emerging diseases. Because influenza exists in the human population in an ever-present but relatively benign form, changing just a little from year to year, we tend, quite mistakenly, to think we understand the nature of the threat that it presents.

Bird Flu cannot be eradicated, we must learn to live with it.

Despite the apparent "novelty" of a strain of bird flu that can sweep across the globe and kill not only the domesticated foul that carries the virus causing the pandemic, but also those humans unfortunate enough to get too close to the sick birds they tend, finding influenza in domesticated birds is not the least bit uncommon.

The natural reservoir for influenza virus is in fact the intestines of water fowl. In particular, ducks habour the virus, and suffer no ill effects from doing so. Because these migratory birds are always on the move, and because they shed virus in the waterways that they inhabit, influenza virus travels widely and is easily transmitted from bird to bird.

Because of this, domesticated birds, like the turkey and the chicken, which cross paths with the virus, become infected and habor the potential to transmit the virus to humans (for example, virus secreted onto the surface of eggs could end up infecting egg handlers— for this reason, if bird handlers notice any of the following symptons in their birds they should immediately notify Federal or State animal health officials: sudden death; lack of energy and appetite; decreased egg production; soft-shelled or misshapen eggs; swelling; purple discoloration; nasal discharge; coughing, sneezing; lack of coordination and diarrhea).

Often an intermediate host, the pig, is involved in the cross-species transmission of influenza. When this happens, the result is referred to as Swine Flu. Even so, the source of the virus is generally aquatic birds.

Most strains of bird flu *do not* cross species and end up infecting humans. However the H5N1 strain that has in the last decade been known to infect humans, and kill them in 5 out of every 10 cases, clearly has surmounted the first of two barriers that must be cleared before a bird flu pandemic can take hold in the human population. The second barrier will be surmounted when this strain acquires the ability to jump from one human to another. This may never happen, and hopefully will not. But based on the history of pandemic flu, it seems more likely that this is just a matter of time. Whether this takes one year or twenty is just impossible to say.

The World Health Organisation has estimated that a human-to-human strain of bird flu could result in an influenza pandemic with the potential to cause between 2 and 7 million fatalities worldwide. Considering the underwhelming state of health services offered by the majority of countries in the world today, these numbers do not appear to be overhyped estimates of the potential lethality of a bird flu pandemic. Should a bird flu pandemic break out with a lethality approaching that of the 1918 Spanish Flu pandemic, it is probably fair to state that the WHO prediction is likely to fall far short of the actual death toll.

Emergence of a Bird Flu Pandemic?

The current candidate for the cause of a bird flu pandemic that crosses into the human population is the H5N1 strain. As discussed in my essay on The 1918 Spanish Flu Pandemic, and the Emerging Bird Flu Pandemic, this strain was first detected in Hong Kong in 1997, and in the time since then has spread halfway across the globe despite strenuous efforts to eradicate it in poultry stocks that have become infected. This movement of the virus, which requires transmission from one (bird) host to another via shared waterways, is slow in comparison to the movement of an airborne strain which can be transmitted from one human host to another in the particulate matter exchanged during coughing and sneezing events. The pandemic of 1918 spread across the globe in about six months, despite the dependence of that time on ship borne travel. In an age of international travel, this encircling time could be reduced to a matter of days. Once it begins, the likelihood that it can be stopped in its tracks is small.

Life during a Bird Flu Pandemic

One can never predict with any accuracy the way a natural catastrophe will unfold. But some speculation on life during the time of a bird flu pandemic seems worthwhile. Things we can say for certain are the following:

No country will be fully prepared for the event. This stems from the fact that no government is ever prepared for any natural catastrophe, as such preparations are prohibitively expensive. This means the bulk of the population will not have access to medical treatment when they need it. Families will be required to look after themselves. Only the patients identified in the very first stages of a bird flu pandemic are likely to receive treatment.

Medical supplies for combating a bird flu pandemic in the human population will be quickly exhausted. Even now, access to such antivirals as Tamiflu is poor in most parts of the world. (In late 2005 the makers of Tamiflu stepped up production to 10 times the normal level in response to worldwide demand for the drug in anticipation of an impending pandemic).

Likewise, flu vaccines, which require a long lead time for preparation (six months or more) and can easily be "spoiled" due to inadequate preparation, will not be available in anything like a sufficient supply in the foreseeable future.

Social disruption will be significant. When workers are faced with the decision of weighing the safety of family members against the worth of their job, you can bet the absentee rate will skyrocket during a pandemic. When the loss of workers begins to affect the delivery of food supplies, power, and water, we are suddenly looking at a different kind of emergency scenario—one reminiscent of the scenes that played out in New Orleans after Hurricane Katrina struck in 2005. When the services we take for granted every day suddenly disappear, people become desparate and things go to hell rather quickly. The break down of social order may be the most frightening prospect that an emerging bird flu pandemic could bring about.

Preparing for a Bird Flu Pandemic

It is tempting for all of us, the author included, to stick our heads in the sand and hope that the news stories about the possibly of an impending *bird flu pandemic* are mostly hype. But this is about as wise as living in Florida and hoping you have seen the last hurricane, or living in Los Angeles and assuming that you'll not be hit by another earthquake. Really it is just a matter of time, though no one knows how much.

There are some not so difficult things you can do to prepare, things that will also help prepare you for other emergency events. These seems practical to me:

Stock up on water. You can never have too much of this in storage, and it is cheap. Have at least a 3 month supply in stock at any time (6 months if practical), and rotate your supply so that you use up the oldest bottles at the rate you replace them with new ones. This way you will never have to worry about filtering existing water supplies if it comes to water shortages in your area.

Stock up on food supplies. This one is a little more difficult, but if you are lucky enough to have one of those huge freezers in your home, fill it up. Rotate your food, so that it is never more than 3 (or 6) months old. Be sure to buy only the foods you normally buy, as you'll be eating them regardless of whether or not any disaster strikes. Dry foods can be stored separately, but people tend too forget about them and only check their supplies in the advent of an emergency. So be prepared to toss these after a year when they are no longer edible.

Purchase some quantity of air filtration masks which, in the event of a true bird flu pandemic will be regarded as indispensible when you need to leave the house and mix with the general populace. As regards what type of mask you should obtain if you are inclined to purchase a box or two (not a bad idea as you won't be able to do it if the time comes that you need to wear them) the Centres for Disease Control and Prevention advise health workers to use a "fit-tested respirator, at least as protective as a National Institute of Occupational Safety and Health (NIOSH)-approved N-95 filtering facepiece (i.e., disposable) respirator" as one of the possible precautions against airborne infection when working with patients with known or suspected SARS or Bird Flu. 3M manufactures such masks, and the latest variety with the "Cool Flow" exhalation valve for increased comfort during extended wearing periods seems to be the mask of choice.

For other possible preparedness items you might check out a Distributor of Flu Preparedness Items (naturally enough!).

If it comes down to it, and an infectious form of bird flu arrives in your country, one of the most important things you can do to avoid infection is practice safe hygiene. This means that you go into obsessive compulsive mode and assume that everything you touch has the potential to be carrying virus. It's somewhat pointless to assume this of the contents of your own home (unless you have a stricken person on site) but once you leave the house, it is a good operating assumption. This means under no circumstances do you touch your hands to your face while in public. Children, and adults, who have the habit of putting their fingers in their eyes and noses are *extremely susceptible* to infection in such an environment. When you return to your home, clothing goes into the laundry immediately and you wash your hands thoroughly with soap to rinse away any virus you might have come in contact with. You always use a face mask in public if you have access to one. Otherwise you make one. Common sense suggests that anything that inhibits the likelihood of inhaled aerosolised influenza is better than nothing. But a proper face mask is designed to be efficient at this task. These are designed to be used *once only* and discarded.

If you are a vendor, think about how you might change the operational nature of your business to stay afloat during a time of crisis. What can you do to reduce the likelihood that your employees will desert you? For instance, if you sell clothing you are very unlikely to receive my business if I must enter an enclosed space (a building) in order to purchase something. At such a time I do not want to breathe the air of a confined space. But if your stock was accessible in an open-air market I would probably be much more inclined. Employees will feel the same way, particularly if the goods in question are not critical to day to day survival.

Finally, do some more reading on the subject of bird flu pandemic. The information about bird flu found on this page is by no means exhaustive. Reading resources are listed below in the Related Links section.

Could a Bird Flu Pandemic resemble the Spanish Flu Pandemic of 1918?

A lot has happened in the last decade as regards our scientific understanding of the genetic mechanisms responsible for the virulence of some strains of influenza. Much of this new understanding has been a direct result of the work of Dr. Jeffery Taubenberger and his team at the Armed Forces Institute of Pathology. Back in 1998 I interviewed Dr. Taubenberger about his effort to reconstruct the genes of the 1918 Spanish Flu virus. At the time I had forseen the day when it would be possible to reconstruct the entire virus.

In October of 2005, after 10 years of work by Taubenberger's team, it was finally reported that the virus had been re-engineered. You can read about the announcement in the PBS article entitled 1918 Spanish Flu Offers Clues About Pandemic Viruses. Of particular interest is the observation that Taubenberger's work "published in the journal Nature in October 2005, offered some parallels between the Spanish flu virus and the H5N1 strain of the bird flu slowly spreading through Asia and recently turning up in other parts of the world." The implication here is clear. If the currently circulating H5N1 bird flu virus does acquire human-to-human transmission, the estimated mortality rates offered by the World Health Organisation for a bird flu pandemic could prove to be wildy optimistic.

Influenza Vaccine

The influenza vaccine, also known as flu shot, is an annual vaccine to protect against the highly variable influenza virus. Each injected seasonal influenza vaccine contains three influenza viruses: one influenza type A subtype H3N2 virus strain, one influenza type A subtype H1N1 (seasonal) virus strain, and one influenza type B virus strain.

Purpose and Benefits of Annual Flu Vaccination

"Influenza vaccination is the most effective method for preventing influenza virus infection and its potentially severe complications."

Deadly Epidemics each Winter

An influenza epidemic emerges during flu season each winter. There are two flu seasons annually, corresponding to the occurrence of winter in opposite months in the Northern and Southern Hemispheres.

Worldwide, seasonal influenza kills an estimated 250,000 to 500,000 people each year. Tens of thousands of Americans die in a typical flu season, but there are notable variations from year to year. In 2010 the Centres for Disease Control and Prevention (CDC) in the United States changed the way it reports the 30 year estimates for deaths from influenza. Now they are reported as a range from a low of about 3,300 deaths to a high of 49,000 per year over the past 30 years.

The majority of deaths in the industrialised world occur in adults aged 65 and over. A review at the NIAID division of the NIH in 2008 concluded that "Seasonal influenza causes more than 200,000 hospitalisations and 41,000 deaths in the U.S. every year, and is the seventh leading cause of death in the U.S." The average total economic costs caused by the annual influenza outbreak in the U.S. have been estimated at over $80 billion.

The number of annual influenza-related hospitalisations is many times the number of deaths. "The high costs of hospitalising young children for influenza creates a significant economic burden in the United States, underscoring the importance of preventive flu shots

for children and the people with whom they have regular contact..."
In 2006 the United States began recommending influenza vaccinations
for preschoolers but Canada did not follow suit until 2010, "thereby
creating a natural experiment to evaluate the effect of the policy in
the United States."

A Canadian study found emergency room visits significantly lower
for 2- to 4 year olds in Boston than in Montreal through the period
(34% fewer ER trips). Vaccination of preschoolers may have reduced
their likelihood of transmission of flu to older siblings and raised the
chances that their parents would vaccinate older children as well,
since there were also 18 percent fewer emergency room visits by 5-
to 18 year olds in Boston than Montreal during the study period.

In another six-year observational study, vaccination of children
aged 6 months through 5 years was found to prevent illness in more
than half.

National Advice on Flu Vaccination

In Canada, the National Advisory Committee on Immunisation,
the group that advises the Public Health Agency of Canada, currently
recommends that everyone aged 2 to 64 years be encouraged to receive
annual influenza vaccination, and that children between the age of
six and 24 months, and their household contacts, should be considered
a high priority for the flu vaccine.

In the United States, "Routine influenza vaccination is
recommended for all persons aged e"6 months." The sole group for
whom routine influenza vaccination is still not recommended is infants
less than six months of age.

Within its blanket recommendation for general vaccination, the
United States, the Centres for Disease Control and Prevention (CDC)
emphasizes to clinicians the special urgency of vaccination for members
of certain vulnerable groups, and their caregivers:

Vaccination is especially important for people at higher risk of
serious influenza complications or people who live with or care for
people at higher risk for serious complications.

Benefits of Vaccination

Vaccination against influenza is also, according to research
published in July 2010, thought to be important for members of high-
risk groups who would be likely to suffer complications from influenza,

for example pregnant women and children and teenagers from six months to 18 years of age; In expanding the new upper age limit to 18 years, the aim is to reduce both the time children and parents lose from visits to pediatricians and missing school and the need for antibiotics for complications.

An added expected benefit would be indirect — to reduce the number of influenza cases among parents and other household members, and possibly spread to the general community.

Vaccination of school-age children has a strong protective effect on the adults and elderly with whom the children are in contact. Children born to mothers who received flu vaccination while pregnant are strongly protected from having to be hospitalised with the flu. "The effectiveness of influenza vaccine given to mothers during pregnancy in preventing hospitalisation among their infants, adjusted for potential confounders, was 91.5%."

Healthy, working adults who received influenza vaccine reported 25 percent fewer episodes of upper respiratory illness than those who received the placebo (105 vs. 140 episodes per 100 subjects, $P < 0.001$), 43 percent fewer days of sick leave from work due to upper respiratory illness (70 vs. 122 days per 100 subjects, $P = 0.001$), and 44 percent fewer visits to physicians' offices for upper respiratory illnesses (31 vs. 55 visits per 100 subjects, $P = 0.004$). The study, reported in the NEJM, estimated cost savings at $46.85 per person vaccinated, and concluded that "Vaccination against influenza has substantial health-related and economic benefits for healthy, working adults."

Influenza vaccination has been shown highly effective in health care workers, with minimal adverse effects. In a study of forty matched nursing homes, staff influenza vaccination rates were 69.9% in the vaccination arm versus 31.8% in the control arm. The vaccinated staff experienced a 42% reduction in sick leave from work ($P=.03$). A review of eighteen studies likewise found a strong net benefit to health care workers. The two of these eighteen studies that assessed the relationship of patient mortality relative to staff influenza vaccine uptake both found that higher rates of health care worker vaccination correlated with reduced patient deaths. An analysis of data and patient population health in New Mexico's 75 long-term care facilities nursing homes found that as vaccination rates of health care personnel with direct patient contact rose from 51 to 75 percent, the chances of a flu outbreak among patients in that facility went down by 87 percent.

The New Mexico study showed that vaccinating health care personnel provided more protection to residents than vaccinating residents themselves.

In a 2010 survey of healthcare workers, 63.5% reported that they received the flu vaccine during the 2010-11 season, an increase from 61.9% reported the previous season. Health professionals with direct patient contact had higher vaccination uptake, such as physicians and dentists (84.2%) and nurse practitioners (82.6%).

Cross-protection

Annual seasonal flu vaccination may provide some level of protection against novel flu viruses. A number of studies suggest that seasonal flu vaccine may offer cross-protection, both against the H5N1-type (avian influenza) H5N1 infection and the 2009 flu pandemic (the H1N1 "swine flu.") Vaccine protection can be long-lasting. Participants who received vaccination against the swine flu in 1976 still enjoyed benefits 33 years later, exhibiting a significantly enhanced immune response to the 2009 pandemic H1N1.

History of the Flu Vaccine

Vaccines are used in both humans and nonhumans. Human vaccine is meant unless specifically identified as a veterinary, poultry or livestock vaccine.

Influenza

The first influenza pandemic was recorded in 1580; since this time, various methods have been employed to eradicate its cause. The etiological cause of influenza, the orthomyxoviridae was finally discovered by the Medical Research Council (MRC) of the United Kingdom in 1933.

Known Flu Pandemics

1889–90 — Asiatic (Russian) Flu, mortality rate said to be 0.75–1 death per 1000 possibly H2N2

1900 — Possibly H3N8

1918–20 – Spanish Flu, 500 million ill, at least 20–40 million died of H1N1

1957–58 – Asian Flu, 1 to 1.5 million died of H2N2

1968–69 – Hong Kong Flu, 3/4 to 1 million died of H3N2

2009 - Swine Flu, caused by H1N1/09, 14,286 died.

Flu Vaccine Origins and Development

In the world wide Spanish flu pandemic of 1918, "Physicians tried everything they knew, everything they had ever heard of, from the ancient art of bleeding patients, to administering oxygen, to developing new vaccines and sera (chiefly against what we now call *Hemophilus influenzae*—a name derived from the fact that it was originally considered the etiological agent—and several types of pneumococci). Only one therapeutic measure, transfusing blood from recovered patients to new victims, showed any hint of success."

In 1931, viral growth in embryonated hens' eggs was reported by Ernest William Goodpasture and colleagues at Vanderbilt University. The work was extended to growth of influenza virus by several workers, including Thomas Frances, Wilson Smith and Macfarlane Burnet, leading to the first experimental influenza vaccines. In the 1940s, the US military developed the first approved inactivated vaccines for influenza, which were used in the Second World War. Greater advances were made in vaccinology and immunology, and vaccines became safer and mass-produced. Today, thanks to the advances of molecular technology, we are on the verge of making influenza vaccines through the genetic manipulation of influenza genes.

Flu Vaccine Acceptance

According to the CDC: "Influenza vaccination is the primary method for preventing influenza and its severe complications. Vaccination is associated with reductions in influenza-related respiratory illness and physician visits among all age groups, hospitalisation and death among persons at high risk, otitis media among children, and work absenteeism among adults. Although influenza vaccination levels increased substantially during the 1990s, further improvements in vaccine coverage levels are needed".

The current egg-based technology for producing influenza vaccine was created in the 1950s. In the U.S. swine flu scare of 1976, President Gerald Ford was confronted with a potential swine flu pandemic. The vaccination program was rushed, yet plagued by delays and public relations problems. Meanwhile, maximum military containment efforts succeeded unexpectedly in confining the new strain to the single army base where it had originated. On that base a number of soldiers fell severely ill, but only one died. The program was cancelled, after about 24% of the population had received vaccinations. An excess in deaths of twenty-five over normal annual levels as well as 400 excess hospitalisations, both from Guillain-Barré syndrome, were estimated to have occurred from the vaccination program itself, illustrating that vaccine itself is not free of risks. The result has been cited to stoke lingering doubts about vaccination. In the end, however, even the maligned 1976 vaccine may have saved lives. A 2010 study found a significantly enhanced immune response against the 2009 pandemic H1N1 in study participants who had received vaccination against the swine flu in 1976.

Current Status

Influenza research includes molecular virology, molecular evolution, pathogenesis, host immune responses, genomics, and epidemiology. These help in developing influenza countermeasures such as vaccines, therapies and diagnostic tools. Improved influenza countermeasures require basic research on how viruses enter cells, replicate, mutate, evolve into new strains and induce an immune response. The Influenza Genome Sequencing Project is creating a library of influenza sequences that will help us understand what makes one strain more lethal than another, what genetic determinants most affect immunogenicity, and how the virus evolves over time. Solutions to limitations in current vaccine methods are being researched.

The rapid development, production, and distribution of pandemic influenza vaccines could potentially save millions of lives during an influenza pandemic. Due to the short time frame between identification of a pandemic strain and need for vaccination, researchers are looking at novel technologies for vaccine production that could provide better "real-time" access and be produced more affordably, thereby increasing access for people living in low- and moderate-income countries, where an influenza pandemic may likely originate, such as live attenuated (egg-based or cell-based) technology and recombinant technologies (proteins and virus-like particles).

As of July 2009, more than 70 known clinical trials have been completed or are ongoing for pandemic influenza vaccines. In September 2009, the US Food and Drug Administration approved four vaccines against the 2009 H1N1 influenza virus (the current pandemic strain), and expected the initial vaccine lots to be available within the following month.

Prospects for Universal Flu Vaccines

Many groups world wide are working on a universal flu vaccine that will not need changing each year, as the sector has been viewed as "increasingly hot". Companies pursuing the vaccine as of 2009 and 2010 include BiondVax, Theraclone, Dynavax Technologies Corporation, VaxInnate, Crucell NV, Inovio Pharmaceuticals, and Immune Targeting Systems (ITS)

In 2008 Acambis announced work on a universal flu vaccine (ACAM-FLU-ATM) based on the less variable M2 protein component of the flu virus shell.

In 2009, the Wistar Institute received a patent for using "a variety of peptides" in a flu vaccine, and announced it was seeking a corporate partner.

In 2010, the National Institute of Allergy and Infectious Diseases (NIAID) of the U.S. NIH announced a breakthrough; the effort targets the stem, which mutates less often than the head of the virus.

DNA vaccines such as VGX-3400X (aimed at multiple H5N1 strains) contain DNA fragments (plasmids). Inovios SynCon DNA vaccines include H5N1 and H1N1 subtypes.

In July 2011, F16 researchers created an antibody, which targets a protein found on the surface of all influenza A viruses called haemagglutinin.

F16 is the only known antibody that treats all 16 subtypes of the influenza A virus and might be the lynchpin for a universal influenza vaccine.

Other Vaccines are Polypeptide Based

Some universal flu vaccines have started early stage clinical trials.

BiondVax are targeting the less variable stalk of the haemagglutinin molecule with Multimeric-001. This is aimed at type A (inc H1N1) and Type B influenza and has started a phase IIa study.

Dynavax have developed a vaccine N8295 based on two highly conserved antigens NP and M2e and their TLR9 agonist, and started clinical trials in June 2010.

ITS's fp01 includes 6 peptide antigens to highly conserved segments of the PA, PB1, PB2, NP & M1 proteins, and has started phase I trials.

Based on the results of animal studies, a universal flu vaccine may use a two-step vaccination strategy — priming with a DNA-based HA vaccine followed by a second dose with an inactivated, attenuated, or adenovirus-vector–based vaccine.

Some people given a 2009 H1N1 flu vaccine have developed broadly protective antibodies which has raised hopes for a universal flu vaccine.

Clinical Trials of Vaccines

A vaccine is assessed by the reduction of the risk of disease that is produced by vaccination, the vaccine's *efficacy*. In contrast, in the field, the *effectiveness* of a vaccine is the practical reduction in risk for an individual when they are vaccinated under real-world conditions. Measuring efficacy of influenza vaccines is relatively simple, as the immune response produced by the vaccine can be assessed in animal models, or the amount of antibody produced in vaccinated people can be measured, or most rigorously, by immunising adult volunteers and then challenging with virulent influenza virus. In studies such as these, influenza vaccines showed high efficacy and produced a protective immune response. For ethical reasons, such challenge studies cannot be performed in the population most at risk from influenza – the elderly and young children. However, studies on the effectiveness of flu vaccines in the real world are uniquely difficult. The vaccine may not be matched to the viruses in circulation that year; virus prevalence varies widely between years, and influenza is often confused with other influenza-like illnesses.

Nevertheless, multiple clinical trials of both live and inactivated influenza vaccines against seasonal influenza have been performed and their results pooled and analysed in several recent meta-analyses. Studies on live vaccines have very limited data, but these preparations may be more effective than inactivated vaccines. The meta-analyses examined the efficacy and effectiveness of inactivated vaccines against seasonal influenza in adults, children, and the elderly. In adults, vaccines show high efficacy against the targeted strains, but low effectiveness overall, so the benefits of vaccination are small, with a one-quarter reduction in risk of contracting influenza but no significant effect on the rate of hospitalisation. However, the risk of serious complications from influenza is small in adults, so unless the effect from vaccination is large it might not have been detected. In children, vaccines again showed high efficacy, but low effectiveness in preventing "flu-like illness". In children under two the data are extremely limited, but vaccination appeared to confer no measurable benefit. In the elderly, vaccination does not reduce the frequency of influenza, but seems to reduce pneumonia, hospital admission and deaths from influenza or pneumonia. However, the current data on the effectiveness of influenza vaccines in the elderly may be unreliable, due to high levels of selection bias.

Overall, the benefit of influenza vaccination is clear in the elderly and vaccination of children may be beneficial. Routine vaccination of adults is not predicted to produce significant improvements in public health. The apparent contradiction between vaccines with high efficacy, but low effectiveness, may reflect the difficulty in diagnosing influenza under clinical conditions and the large number of strains circulating in the population. In contrast, during an influenza pandemic, where a single strain of virus is responsible for illnesses, an effective vaccine could produce a large decrease in the number of cases and be highly effective in controlling an epidemic. However, such a vaccine would have to be produced and distributed rapidly to have maximum effect.

Effectiveness of Vaccine

The CDC reports that studies demonstrate that vaccination is a cost-effective counter-measure to seasonal outbreaks of influenza. However it is not perfect. A study led by Dr. David K. Shay in February, 2008 reported that:

> *"full immunisation against flu provided about a 75 percent effectiveness rate in preventing hospitalisations from influenza complications in the 2005-6 and 2006-7 influenza seasons."*

Influenza vaccine has been demonstrated to prevent disease and death, both in numerous controlled studies and in painstaking scientific reviews of these studies. However the rigor of the science of these studies has also been criticized. A 2006 Cochrane review of influenza vaccination in the elderly stated "The apparent high effectiveness of the vaccines in preventing death from all causes may reflect a baseline imbalance in health status and other systematic differences in the two groups of participants. In one observational study, a sharply lower risk of death or hospitalisation for pneumonia was seen in vaccinated persons:

Results: The relative risk of death for vaccinated persons compared with unvaccinated persons was 0.39 [95% confidence interval (95% CI), 0.33-0.47] before influenza season, 0.56 (0.52-0.61) during influenza season, and 0.74 (0.67-0.80) after influenza season. The relative risk of pneumonia hospitalisation was 0.72 (0.59-0.89) before, 0.82 (0.75-0.89) during, and 0.95 (0.85-1.07) after influenza season. Adjustment for diagnosis code variables resulted in estimates that were further from the null, in all time periods.

A better vitality and lower pneumonia hospitalisation was thus observed in the vaccinated group in this non-randomised population study before, during, and after influenza season. This could, however, have been ascribed in whole or in part to self-selection bias, since vaccinated persons were already healthier before flu season. Some sub-populations have been assumed to benefit from vaccination in the absence of directly specific studies. For example, a 2008 Cochrane review of healthy children found "Influenza vaccines are efficacious in children older than two but little evidence is available for children under two.". The CDC in 2010, after a review of extant studies, extended its guidelines to recommend that every child over 6 months be given the influenza vaccine. Vaccines were shown effective against the influenza strains they are designed to protect against, but this translated to only a modest impact on working days lost due to influenza-like infections in a 2007 Cochrane review on influenza vaccines in healthy adults. While a 2010 Cochrane review noted that "Influenza vaccines have a modest effect in reducing influenza symptoms and working days lost" it stated found no evidence of prevention of complications, such as pneumonia, or transmission.

The group most vulnerable to non-pandemic flu, the elderly, is also the least benefitted by the vaccine, with an average efficacy rate ranging from 40-50% at age 65, and only 15-30% past age 70. There are multiple reasons behind this steep decline in vaccine efficacy, the most common of which are the declining immunological function and frailty associated with advanced age. An influenza vaccine with four times the usual amount of antigen (Fluzone High Dose) has shown increased immune response in the elderly and has now been approved by the U.S. Food and Drug Administration (FDA).

In a non-pandemic year, a person in the United States aged 50–64 is nearly ten times more likely to die an influenza-associated death than a younger person, and a person over age 65 is over ten times more likely to die an influenza-associated death than the 50–64 age group. Vaccination of those over age 65 reduces influenza-associated death by about 50%. However, it is unlikely that the vaccine completely explains the results since elderly people who get vaccinated are probably more healthy and health-conscious than those who do not. Elderly participants randomised to a high-dose group (60 micrograms) had antibody levels 44 to 79 percent higher than did those who received the normal dose of vaccine. Elderly volunteers receiving the higher dose were more likely to achieve protective levels of antibody.

As mortality is also high among infants who contract influenza, the household contacts and caregivers of infants should be vaccinated to reduce the risk of passing an influenza infection to the infant. Data from the years when Japan required annual flu vaccinations for school-aged children indicate that vaccinating children the group most likely to catch and spread the disease—has a strikingly positive effect on reducing mortality among older people: one life saved for every 420 children who received the flu vaccine.

This may be due to herd immunity or to direct causes, such as individual older people not being exposed to influenza. For example, retired grandparents often risk infection by caring for their sick grandchildren in households where the parents can't take time off work or are sick themselves.

In most years (16 of the 19 years before 2007), the flu vaccine strains have been a good match for the circulating strains. In other flu seasons like that of 2007/2008, the match was less useful. But even a mismatched vaccine can often provide some protection:

Antibodies made in response to vaccination with one strain of influenza viruses can provide protection against different, but related strains. A less than ideal match may result in reduced vaccine effectiveness against the variant viruses, but it still can provide enough protection to prevent or lessen illness severity and prevent flu-related complications.

In addition, it's important to remember that the influenza vaccine contains three virus strains so the vaccine can also protect against the other two viruses. For these reasons, even during seasons when there is a less than ideal match, CDC continues to recommend influenza vaccination. This is particularly important for people at high risk for serious flu complications and their close contacts.

Comparing Flu Shot to Nasal Spray

Flu vaccines are available either as:

TIV (flu shot (injection) of trivalent (three strains; usually A/H1N1, A/H3N2, and B) inactivated (killed) vaccine) or

LAIV (nasal spray (mist) of live attenuated influenza vaccine.)

TIV works by putting into the bloodstream those parts of three strains of flu virus that the body uses to create antibodies; while LAIV works by inoculating against those same three strains that have been genetically modified to minimise symptoms of illness.

LAIV is not recommended for individuals under age 2 or over age 50, but might be comparatively more effective among children over age 2.

A military study on military personnel showed that flu shots yielded less illness than nasal spray. Based on one of the largest head-to-head studies comparing LAIV and TIV (which was conducted by the U.S. Armed Forces Surveillance Centre on military personnel who were stationed in the United States during three flu seasons from 2004 through 2007), investigators concluded that: "It may be prudent to use TIV in patients who were vaccinated at least once in the past 2 years but LAIV against pandemic strains may be more protective than inactivated vaccines, because the population will probably lack preexisting immunity."

High-dose Vaccine

A high-dose vaccine (Fluzone High-Dose) 4x the strength of standard flu vaccine was approved by the FDA in late 2009. This vaccine is intended for people 65 and over, who typically have weakened immune response due to normal aging.

The vaccine produces a greater immune response than standard vaccine, but it is not yet known whether it provides greater protection against flu. Study results are expected in 2012. CDC recommends the high-dose vaccine for people 65 and over but expresses no preference between it and standard vaccine.

Vaccination Recommendations

Various public health organisations, including the World Health Organisation, have recommended that yearly influenza vaccination be routinely offered to patients at risk of complications of influenza and those individuals who live with or care for high-risk individuals, including:

- the elderly (UK recommendation is those aged 65 or above)
- patients with chronic lung diseases (asthma, COPD, etc.)
- patients with chronic heart diseases (congenital heart disease, chronic heart failure, ischaemic heart disease)
- patients with chronic liver diseases (including cirrhosis)
- patients with chronic renal diseases (such as the nephrotic syndrome)
- patients who are immunosuppressed (those with HIV or who are receiving drugs to suppress the immune system such as chemotherapy and long-term steroids) and their household contacts
- people who live together in large numbers in an environment where influenza can spread rapidly, such as prisons, nursing homes, schools, and dormitories
- healthcare workers (both to prevent sickness and to prevent spread to patients)
- pregnant women. However, a 2009 review concluded that there was insufficient evidence to recommend routine use of trivalent influenza vaccine during the first trimester of pregnancy.
- children from ages six months to two years.

Both types of flu vaccines are contraindicated for those with severe allergies to egg proteins and people with a history of Guillain-Barré syndrome.

Public Health Law Research, an independent organisation, published in 2009 several evidence briefs summarising the research assessing the effect of specific laws and policy on public health.

There is sufficient evidence supporting the effectiveness of requiring vaccinations as a condition for attending child care facilities and schools. There is insufficient evidence to assess the effectiveness of requiring vaccinations as a condition for specified jobs as a means of reducing incidence of specific diseases among particularly vulnerable populations.

There is strong evidence supporting the effectiveness of standing orders which allow healthcare workers without prescription authority to administer vaccines under defined circumstances as a public health intervention aimed at increasing vaccination rates.

Side effects

- Side effects of the inactivated/dead flu vaccine injection include:
- mild soreness, redness, and swelling where the shot was given
- fever
- aches
- These problems usually begin soon after the injection, and last 1–2 days.
- Side effects of the activated/live/LAIV flu nasal spray vaccine:
- Some children and adolescents 2–17 years of age have reported:
- runny nose, nasal congestion or cough
- fever
- headache and muscle aches
- wheesing
- abdominal pain or occasional vomiting or diarrhea
- Some adults 18–49 years of age have reported:
- runny nose or nasal congestion
- sore throat
- cough, chills, tiredness/weakness
- headache
- More severe, but very rare side effects include:
- life-threatening allergic reaction.

Some injection-based flu vaccines intended for adults in the United States contain thiomersal (also known as thimerosal). Despite some controversy in the media, the World Health Organisation has concluded that there is no evidence of toxicity from thiomersal in vaccines and no reason on grounds of safety to change to more-expensive single-dose administration.

Although Guillain-Barré syndrome had been feared as a complication of vaccination, the CDC states that most studies on modern influenza vaccines have seen no link with Guillain-Barré.

A review has concluded that the 2009 H1N1 ("swine flu") vaccine has a safety profile similar to that of seasonal vaccine. Although one review gives an incidence of about one case per million vaccinations, a large study in China, reported in the NEJM covering close to 100 million doses of vaccine against the 2009 H1N1 "swine" flu found only eleven cases of Guillain-Barre syndrome, (0.1%) total incidence in persons vaccinated, actually lower than the normal rate of the disease in China, and no other notable side effects; "The risk-benefit ratio, which is what vaccines and everything in medicine is about, is overwhelmingly in favour of vaccination." Getting infected by influenza itself increases both the risk of death (up to 1 in 10,000) and increases the risk of developing Guillain-Barré syndrome to a much higher level than the highest level of suspected vaccine involvement (approx. 10 times higher by recent estimates).

Flu Vaccine Manufacturing

Flu vaccine is usually grown in fertilised chicken eggs. In February preceding each fall's flu season (in the Northern hemisphere), three strains of flu are selected and chicken eggs inoculated.

As of November 2007, both the conventional injection and the nasal spray are manufactured using chicken eggs. The European Union has also approved Optaflu, a vaccine produced by Novartis using vats of animal cells. This technique is expected to be more scalable and avoid problems with eggs, such as allergic reactions and incompatibility with strains that affect avians like chickens. A DNA-based vaccination, which is hoped to be even faster to manufacture, is currently in clinical trials, but has not yet been proven safe and effective. Research continues into the idea of a "universal" influenza vaccine (but no vaccine candidates have been announced) which would not need to be tailored to work on particular strains, but would be effective against a broad variety of influenza viruses.

In a 2007 report, the current global capacity of approximately 826 million seasonal influenza vaccine doses (inactivated and live) was double the current production of 413 million doses. In an aggressive scenario of producing pandemic influenza vaccines by 2013, only 2.8 billion courses could be produced in a six-month time frame. If all high- and upper-middle-income countries sought vaccines for their entire populations in a pandemic, nearly 2 billion courses would be required. If China pursued this goal as well, more than 3 billion courses would be required to serve these populations. Vaccine research and development is ongoing to identify novel vaccine approaches that could produce much greater quantities of vaccine at a price that is affordable to the global population.

An effective method of vaccine generation that bypasses the need for eggs is the construction of "influenza virus-like particle (VLP)". VLP is a non-egg, non-mammalian cell culture-based vaccine, purified from the supernatants of Spodoptera frugiperda Sf9 insect cells following infection of baculovirus vectors encoding an expression cassette made up of only three influenza virus structural proteins, hemagglutinin (HA), neuraminidase (NA), and matrix (M1) VLPs elicit antibodies that recognise a broader panel of antigenically distinct viral isolates compared to other vaccines in the hemagglutination-inhibition (HAI) assay.

H5N1

Vaccines have been formulated against several of the avian H5N1 influenza varieties. Vaccination of poultry against the ongoing H5N1 epizootic is widespread in certain countries. Some vaccines also exist for use in humans, and others are in testing, but none have been made available to civilian populations, nor produced in quantities sufficient to protect more than a tiny fraction of the Earth's population in the event of an H5N1 pandemic.

- Three H5N1 vaccines for humans have been licensed as of June 2008:
- Sanofi Pasteur's vaccine approved by the United States in April 2007,
- GlaxoSmithKline's vaccine Pandemrix approved by the European Union in May 2008, and
- CSL Limited's vaccine approved by Australia in June 2008.
- All are produced in eggs and would require many months to be altered to a pandemic version.

H5N1 continually mutates, meaning vaccines based on current samples of avian H5N1 cannot be depended upon to work in the case of a future pandemic of H5N1. While there can be some cross-protection against related flu strains, the best protection would be from a vaccine specifically produced for any future pandemic flu virus strain. Dr. Daniel Lucey, co-director of the Biohazardous Threats and Emerging Diseases graduate program at Georgetown University, has made this point, "There is no H5N1 pandemic so there can be no pandemic vaccine." However, "pre-pandemic vaccines" have been created; are being refined and tested; and do have some promise both in furthering research and preparedness for the next pandemic. Vaccine manufacturing companies are being encouraged to increase capacity so that if a pandemic vaccine is needed, facilities will be available for rapid production of large amounts of a vaccine specific to a new pandemic strain.

Problems with H5N1 vaccine production include:

- lack of overall production capacity
- lack of surge production capacity (it is impractical to develop a system that depends on hundreds of millions of 11 day old specialised eggs on a standby basis)
- the pandemic H5N1 might be lethal to chickens.

Cell culture (cell-based) manufacturing technology can be applied to influenza vaccines as they are with most viral vaccines and thereby solve the problems associated with creating flu vaccines using chicken eggs as is currently done.:

Currently, influenza vaccine for the annual, seasonal influenza program comes from four manufacturers. However, only a single manufacturer produces the annual vaccine entirely within the U.S. Thus, if a pandemic occurred and existing U.S.-based influenza vaccine manufacturing capacity was completely diverted to producing a pandemic vaccine, supply would be severely limited. Moreover, because the annual influenza manufacturing process takes place during most of the year, the time and capacity to produce vaccine against potential pandemic viruses for a stockpile, while continuing annual influenza vaccine production, is limited. Since supply will be limited, it is critical for HHS to be able to direct vaccine distribution in accordance with predefined groups; HHS will ensure the building of capacity and will engage states in a discussion about the purchase and distribution of pandemic influenza vaccine.

Vaccine production capacity: The protective immune response generated by current influenza vaccines is largely based on viral hemagglutinin (HA) and neuraminidase (NA) antigens in the vaccine. As a consequence, the basis of influenza vaccine manufacturing is growing massive quantities of virus in order to have sufficient amounts of these protein antigens to stimulate immune responses. Influenza vaccines used in the United States and around world are manufactured by growing virus in fertilised hens' eggs, a commercial process that has been in place for decades. To achieve current vaccine production targets millions of 11-day old fertilised eggs must be available every day of production.

In the near term, further expansion of these systems will provide additional capacity for the U.S.-based production of both seasonal and pandemic vaccines, however, the surge capacity that will be needed for a pandemic response cannot be met by egg-based vaccine production alone, as it is impractical to develop a system that depends on hundreds of millions of 11-day old specialised eggs on a standby basis. In addition, because a pandemic could result from an avian influenza strain that is lethal to chickens, it is impossible to ensure that eggs will be available to produce vaccine when needed.

In contrast, cell culture manufacturing technology can be applied to influenza vaccines as they are with most viral vaccines (e.g., polio vaccine, measles-mumps-rubella vaccine, chickenpox vaccine). In this system, viruses are grown in closed systems such as bioreactors containing large numbers of cells in growth media rather than eggs. The surge capacity afforded by cell-based technology is insensitive to seasons and can be adjusted to vaccine demand, as capacity can be increased or decreased by the number of bioreactors or the volume used within a bioreactor. In addition to supporting basic research on cell-based influenza vaccine development, HHS is currently supporting a number of vaccine manufacturers in the advanced development of cell-based influenza vaccines with the goal of developing U.S.-licensed cell-based influenza vaccines produced in the United States. The US government has purchased from Sanofi Pasteur and Chiron Corporation several million doses of vaccine meant to be used in case of an influenza pandemic of H5N1 avian influenza and is conducting clinical trials with these vaccines. Researchers at the University of Pittsburgh have had success with a genetically engineered vaccine that took only a month to make and completely protected chickens from the highly pathogenic H5N1 virus.

According to the United States Department of Health & Human Services

In addition to supporting basic research on cell-based influenza vaccine development, HHS is currently supporting a number of vaccine manufacturers in the advanced development of cell-based influenza vaccines with the goal of developing U.S.-licensed cell-based influenza vaccines produced in the United States. Dose-sparing technologies. Current U.S.-licensed vaccines stimulate an immune response based on the quantity of HA (hemagglutinin) antigen included in the dose. Methods to stimulate a strong immune response using less HA antigen are being studied in H5N1 and H9N2 vaccine trials. These include changing the mode of delivery from intramuscular to intradermal and the addition of immune-enhancing adjuvant to the vaccine formulation. Additionally, HHS is soliciting contract proposals from manufacturers of vaccines, adjuvants, and medical devices for the development and licensure of influenza vaccines that will provide dose-sparing alternative strategies.

Chiron Corporation is now recertified and under contract with the National Institutes of Health to produce 8,000–10,000 investigational doses of Avian Flu (H5N1) vaccine. MedImmune and Aventis Pasteur are under similar contracts. The United States government hopes to obtain enough vaccine in 2006 to treat 4 million people. However, it is unclear whether this vaccine would be effective against a hypothetical mutated strain that would be easily transmitted through human populations, and the shelflife of stockpiled doses has yet to be determined.

The *New England Journal of Medicine* reported on March 30, 2006 on one of dozens of vaccine studies currently being conducted. The Treanor et al. study was on vaccine produced from the human isolate (A/Vietnam/1203/2004 H5N1) of a virulent clade 1 influenza A (H5N1) virus with the use of a plasmid rescue system, with only the hemagglutinin and neuraminidase genes expressed and administered without adjuvant. "The rest of the genes were derived from an avirulent egg-adapted influenza A/PR/8/34 strain. The hemagglutinin gene was further modified to replace six basic amino acids associated with high pathogenicity in birds at the cleavage site between hemagglutinin 1 and hemagglutinin 2. Immunogenicity was assessed by microneutralisation and hemagglutination-inhibition assays with the use of the vaccine virus, although a subgroup of samples were tested with the use of the wild-type influenza A/Vietnam/ 1203/2004 (H5N1) virus." The results of this study combined with others scheduled to be completed by spring 2007 is hoped will provide a highly immunogenic vaccine that is cross-protective against heterologous influenza strains.

On August 18, 2006. the World Health Organisation changed the H5N1 strains recommended for candidate vaccines for the first time since 2004. "The WHO's new prototype strains, prepared by reverse genetics, include three new H5N1 subclades. The hemagglutinin sequences of most of the H5N1 avian influenza viruses circulating in the past few years fall into two genetic groups, or clades. Clade 1 includes human and bird isolates from Vietnam, Thailand, and Cambodia and bird isolates from Laos and Malaysia. Clade 2 viruses were first identified in bird isolates from China, Indonesia, Japan, and South Korea before spreading westward to the Middle East, Europe, and Africa. The clade 2 viruses have been primarily responsible for human H5N1 infections that have occurred during late 2005 and 2006, according to WHO. Genetic analysis has identified six subclades of clade 2, three of which have a distinct geographic distribution and have been implicated in human infections:

- Subclade 1, Indonesia
- Subclade 2, Middle East, Europe, and Africa
- Subclade 3, China

On the basis of the three subclades, the WHO is offering companies and other groups that are interested in pandemic vaccine development these three new prototype strains:

- An A/Indonesia/2/2005-like virus
- An A/Bar headed goose/Quinghai/1A/2005-like virus
- An A/Anhui/1/2005-like virus.

Until now, researchers have been working on prepandemic vaccines for H5N1 viruses in clade 1. In March, the first clinical trial of a U.S. vaccine for H5N1 showed modest results. In May, French researchers showed somewhat better results in a clinical trial of an H5N1 vaccine that included an adjuvant. Vaccine experts aren't sure if a vaccine effective against known H5N1 viral strains would be effective against future strains. Although the new viruses will now be available for vaccine research, WHO said clinical trials using the clade 1 viruses should continue as an essential step in pandemic preparedness, because the trials yield useful information on priming, cross-reactivity, and cross-protection by vaccine viruses from different clades and subclades."

As of November 2006, the United States Department of Health and Human Services still had enough H5N1 pre-pandemic vaccine to treat about 3 million people (5.9 million full-potency doses) in spite of 0.2 million doses used for research and 1.4 million doses that have begun to lose potency (from the original 7.5 million full-potency doses purchased from Sanofi Pasteur and Chiron Corp.). The expected shelf life of seasonal flu vaccine is about a year so the fact that most of the H5N1 pre-pandemic stockpile is still good after about 2 years is considered encouraging.

Annual Reformulation of Flu Vaccine

Each year, three strains are chosen for selection in that year's flu vaccination by the WHO Global Influenza Surveillance Network. The chosen strains are the H1N1, H3N2, and Type-B strains thought most likely to cause significant human suffering in the coming season. Due to the high mutation rate of the virus a particular vaccine formulation is effective for at most about a year. The World Health Organisation coordinates the contents of the vaccine each year to contain the most likely strains of the virus to attack the next year.

"The WHO Global Influenza Surveillance Network was established in 1952. The network comprises 4 WHO Collaborating Centres (WHO CCs) and 112 institutions in 83 countries, which are recognised by WHO as WHO National Influenza Centres (NICs). These NICs collect specimens in their country, perform primary virus isolation and preliminary antigenic characterisation. They ship newly isolated strains to WHO CCs for high level antigenic and genetic analysis, the result of which forms the basis for WHO recommendations on the composition of influenza vaccine for the Northern and Southern Hemisphere each year."

The Global Influenza Surveillance Network's selection of viruses for the vaccine manufacturing process is based on its best estimate of which strains will be predominant the next year, amounting in the end to well-informed but fallible guesswork. Formal WHO recommendations first issued in 1973; beginning 1999 there have been two recommendations per year, one for the northern hemisphere (N) and the other for the southern hemisphere (S).

History of past WHO seasonal influenza vaccine composition recommendations:

2002–2003 Northern Hemisphere Winter Season

The vaccines produced for the 2002–2003 season use:
- an A/New Caledonia/20/1999-like(H1N1);

- an A/Moscow/10/1999-like(H3N2);
- a B/Hong Kong/330/2001-like viruses.

2003 Southern Hemisphere Winter Season

The composition of influenza virus vaccines for use in the 2003 Southern Hemisphere influenza season recommended by the World Health Organisation was:

- an A/New Caledonia/20/99(H1N1)-like virus
- an A/Moscow/10/99(H3N2)-like virus (The widely used vaccine strain is A/Panama/2007/99)
- a B/Hong Kong/330/2001-like virus (Some vaccine strains used were B/Shandong/7/97, B/Hong Kong/330/2001, B/Hong Kong/1434/2002).

2003–2004 Northern Hemisphere Winter Season

The production of flu vaccine requires a lead time of about six months before the season. It is possible that by flu season a strain becomes common for which the vaccine does not provide protection. In the 2003–2004 season the vaccine was produced to protect against A/Panama, A/New Caledonia, and B/Hong Kong. A new strain, A/Fujian, was discovered after production of the vaccine started and vaccination gave only partial protection against this strain.

Nature magazine reported that the Influenza Genome Sequencing Project, using phylogenetic analysis of 156 H3N2 genomes, "explains the appearance, during the 2003–2004 season, of the 'Fujian/411/2002'-like strain, for which the existing vaccine had limited effectiveness" as due to an epidemiologically significant reassortment. "Through a reassortment event, a minor clade provided the haemagglutinin gene that later became part of the dominant strain after the 2002–2003 season. Two of our samples, A/New York/269/2003 (H3N2) and A/New York/32/2003 (H3N2), show that this minor clade continued to circulate in the 2003–2004 season, when most other isolates were reassortants."

According to the CDC

During the 2003–2004 influenza season, influenza A (H1), A (H3N2), and B viruses co-circulated worldwide, and influenza A (H3N2) viruses predominated. Several Asian countries reported widespread outbreaks of avian influenza A (H5N1) among poultry. In Vietnam and Thailand, these outbreaks were associated with severe illnesses and deaths among humans. In the United States, the 2003–2004 influenza season began earlier than most seasons, peaked in December, was moderately severe in terms of its impact on mortality, and was associated predominantly with influenza A (H3N2) viruses.

During September 28, 2003 – May 22, 2004, WHO and NREVSS collaborating laboratories in the United States tested 130,577 respiratory specimens for influenza viruses; 24,649 (18.9%) were positive. Of these, 24,393 (99.0%) were influenza A viruses, and 249 (1.0%) were influenza B viruses. Among the influenza A viruses, 7,191 (29.5%) were subtyped; 7,189 (99.9%) were influenza A (H3N2) viruses, and two (0.1%) were influenza A (H1) viruses. The proportion of specimens testing positive for influenza first increased to >10% during the week ending October 25, 2003 (week 43), peaked at 35.2% during the week ending November 29 (week 48), and declined to <10% during the week ending January 17, 2004 (week 2). The peak percentage of specimens testing positive for influenza during the previous four seasons had ranged from 23% to 31% and peaked during late December to late February.

As of June 15, 2004, CDC had antigenically characterised 1,024 influenza viruses collected by U.S. laboratories since October 1, 2003: 949 influenza A (H3N2) viruses, three influenza A (H1) viruses, one influenza A (H7N2) virus, and 71 influenza B viruses. Of the 949 influenza A (H3N2) isolates characterised, 106 (11.2%) were similar antigenically to the vaccine strain A/Panama/2007/99 (H3N2), and 843 (88.8%) were similar to the drift variant, A/Fujian/411/2002 (H3N2). Of the three A (H1) isolates that were characterised, two were H1N1 viruses, and one was an H1N2 virus. The hemagglutinin proteins of the influenza A (H1) viruses were similar antigenically to the hemagglutinin of the vaccine strain A/New Caledonia/20/99. Of the 71 influenza B isolates that were characterised, 66 (93%) belonged to the B/Yamagata/16/88 lineage and were similar antigenically to B/Sichuan/379/99, and five (7%) belonged to the B/Victoria/2/87 lineage and were similar antigenically to the corresponding vaccine strain B/Hong Kong/330/2001.

H9N2

In December 2003, one confirmed case of avian influenza A (H9N2) virus infection was reported in a child aged five years in Hong Kong.

The child had fever, cough, and nasal discharge in late November, was hospitalised for two days, and fully recovered. The source of this child's H9N2 infection is unknown.

H5N1

During January–March 2004, a total of 34 confirmed human cases of avian influenza A (H5N1) virus infection were reported in Vietnam and Thailand. The cases were associated with severe respiratory illness requiring hospitalisation and a case-fatality proportion of 68% (Vietnam: 22 cases, 15 deaths; Thailand: 12 cases, eight deaths). A substantial proportion of the cases were among children and young adults (i.e., persons aged 5–24 years). These cases were associated with widespread outbreaks of highly pathogenic H5N1 influenza among domestic poultry.

H7N3

During March 2004, health authorities in Canada reported two confirmed cases of avian influenza A (H7N3) virus infection in poultry workers who were involved in culling of poultry during outbreaks of highly pathogenic H7N3 on farms in the Fraser River Valley, British Columbia. One patient had unilateral conjunctivitis and nasal discharge, and the other had unilateral conjunctivitis and headache. Both illnesses resolved without hospitalisation.

H7N2

During the 2003–2004 influenza season, a case of avian influenza A (H7N2) virus infection was detected in an adult male from New York, who was hospitalised for upper and lower respiratory tract illness in November 2003. Influenza A (H7N2) virus was isolated from a respiratory specimen from the patient, whose acute symptoms resolved. The source of this person's infection is unknown.

2004 Southern Hemisphere Winter Season

The composition of influenza virus vaccines for use in the 2004 Southern Hemisphere influenza season recommended by the World Health Organisation was:

- an A/New Caledonia/20/99(H1N1)-like virus
- an A/Fujian/411/2002(H3N2)-like virus (A/Kumamoto/102/2002 and A/Wyoming/3/2003 were egg-grown A/Fujian/411/2002-like viruses)

- a B/Hong Kong/330/2001-like virus (B/Shandong/7/97, B/Hong Kong/330/2001 and B/Hong Kong/1434/2002 were among those used at the time. B/Brisbane/32/2002 was also available.)

2004–2005 Northern Hemisphere Winter Season

On the basis of antigenic analyses of recently isolated influenza viruses, epidemiologic data, and postvaccination serologic studies in humans, the Food and Drug Administration's Vaccines and Related Biological Products Advisory Committee (VRBPAC) recommended that the 2004–05 trivalent influenza vaccine for the United States contain A/New Caledonia/20/99-like (H1N1), A/Fujian/411/2002-like (H3N2), and B/Shanghai/361/2002-like viruses. Because of the growth properties of the A/Wyoming/3/2003 and B/Jiangsu/10/2003 viruses, U.S. vaccine manufacturers are using these antigenically equivalent strains in the vaccine as the H3N2 and B components, respectively. The A/New Caledonia/20/99 virus will be retained as the H1N1 component of the vaccine.

2005 Southern Hemisphere Winter Season

The composition of influenza virus vaccines for use in the 2005 Southern Hemisphere influenza season recommended by the World Health Organisation was:

- an A/New Caledonia/20/99(H1N1)-like virus;
- an A/Wellington/1/2004(H3N2)-like virus;
- a B/Shanghai/361/2002-like virus (B/Shanghai/361/2002, B/Jilin/20/2003 and B/Jiangsu/10/2003 were used at the time)

2005–2006 Northern Hemisphere Winter Season

The vaccines produced for the 2005–2006 season use:

- an A/New Caledonia/20/1999-like(H1N1);
- an A/California/7/2004-like(H3N2) (or the antigenically equivalent strain A/New York/55/2004);
- a B/Jiangsu/10/2003-like viruses.

In people in the United States, overall flu and pneumonia deaths were below those of a typical flu season with 84% Influenzavirus A and the rest Influenzavirus B. Of the patients who had Type A viruses, 80% had viruses identical or similar to the A bugs in the vaccine. 70% of the people testing positive for a B virus had Type B Victoria, a version not found in the vaccine.

"During the 2005–06 season, influenza A (H3N2) viruses predominated overall, but late in the season influenza B viruses were more frequently isolated than influenza A viruses. Influenza A (H1N1) viruses circulated at low levels throughout the season. Nationally, activity was low from October through early January, increased during February, and peaked in early March. Peak activity was less intense, but activity remained elevated for a longer period of time this season compared to the previous three seasons. The longer period of elevated activity may be due in part to regional differences in the timing of peak activity and intensity of influenza B activity later in the season."

2006 Southern Hemisphere Winter Season

The composition of influenza virus vaccines for use in the 2006 Southern Hemisphere influenza season recommended by the World Health Organisation was:

- an A/New Caledonia/20/99(H1N1)-like virus;
- an A/California/7/2004(H3N2)-like virus (A/New York/55/2004 was used at the time);
- a B/Malaysia/2506/2004-like virus.

2006–2007 Northern Hemisphere Winter Season

The 2006–2007 influenza vaccine composition recommended by the World Health Organisation on February 15, 2006 and the U.S. FDA's Vaccines and Related Biological Products Advisory Committee (VRBPAC) on February 17, 2006 use:

- an A/New Caledonia/20/99 (H1N1)-like virus;
- an A/Wisconsin/67/2005 (H3N2)-like virus (A/Wisconsin/67/2005 and A/Hiroshima/52/2005 strains);
- a B/Malaysia/2506/2004-like virus from B/Malaysia/2506/2004 and B/Ohio/1/2005 strains which are of B/Victoria/2/87 lineage.

2007 Southern Hemisphere Winter Season

The composition of influenza virus vaccines for use in the 2007 Southern Hemisphere influenza season recommended by the World Health Organisation on September 20, 2006 was:

- an A/New Caledonia/20/99(H1N1)-like virus,
- an A/Wisconsin/67/2005(H3N2)-like virus (A/Wisconsin/67/2005 and A/Hiroshima/52/2005 were used at the time),
- a B/Malaysia/2506/2004-like virus.

2007–2008 Northern Hemisphere Winter Season

The composition of influenza virus vaccines for use in the 2007–2008 Northern Hemisphere influenza season recommended by the World Health Organisation on February 14, 2007 was:

- an A/Solomon Islands/3/2006 (H1N1)-like virus;
- an A/Wisconsin/67/2005 (H3N2)-like virus (A/Wisconsin/67/2005 (H3N2) and A/Hiroshima/52/2005 were used at the time);
- a B/Malaysia/2506/2004-like virus.

In the US, the CDC reported in Feb 2008 that the H1N1 component was a good match (96%) to the infections occurring. But 87% of the H3N2 are A/Brisbane/10/2007-like viruses, which are a recent antigenic variant of the vaccine strain, A/Wisconsin.

And 93% of the B viruses are in a B/Yamagata lineage that is relatively distinct from the vaccine strain B/Victoria lineage. Only one of the three components was a good match; A/Wisconsin is moderately protective against the drifted A/Brisbane strain. 4.5% of those viruses tested are resistant to Oseltamivir, or Tamiflu—a significant increase over previous years.

This vaccine has been described as 40% effective compared to other years that have been 85–95% effective.

2008 Southern Hemisphere Winter Season

The composition of virus vaccines for use in the 2008 Southern Hemisphere influenza season recommended by the World Health Organisation on September 17–19, 2007 was:

- an A/Solomon Islands/3/2006 (H1N1)-like virus;
- an A/Brisbane/10/2007 (H3N2)-like virus;
- a B/Florida/4/2006-like virus

2008-2009 Northern Hemisphere Winter Season

The composition of virus vaccines for use in the 2008-2009 Northern Hemisphere influenza season recommended by the World Health Organisation on February 14, 2008 was:

- an A/Brisbane/59/2007 (H1N1)-like virus;
- an A/Brisbane/10/2007 (H3N2)-like virus;
- a B/Florida/4/2006-like virus (B/Florida/4/2006 and B/Brisbane/3/2007 (a B/Florida/4/2006-like virus) were used at the time).

As of May 30, 2009: "CDC has antigenically characterised 1,567 seasonal human influenza viruses [947 influenza A (H1), 162 influenza A (H3) and 458 influenza B viruses] collected by U.S. laboratories since October 1, 2008, and 84 novel influenza A (H1N1) viruses. All 947 influenza seasonal A (H1) viruses are related to the influenza A (H1N1) component of the 2008-09 influenza vaccine (A/Brisbane/59/2007). All 162 influenza A (H3N2) viruses are related to the A (H3N2) vaccine component (A/Brisbane/10/2007). All 84 novel influenza A (H1N1) viruses are related to the A/California/07/2009 (H1N1) reference virus selected by WHO as a potential candidate for novel influenza A (H1N1) vaccine. Influenza B viruses currently circulating can be divided into two distinct lineages represented by the B/Yamagata/16/88 and B/Victoria/02/87 viruses. Sixty-one influenza B viruses tested belong to the B/Yamagata lineage and are related to the vaccine strain (B/Florida/04/2006). The remaining 397 viruses belong to the B/Victoria lineage and are not related to the vaccine strain."

2009 Southern Hemisphere Winter Season

The composition of virus vaccines for use in the 2009 Southern Hemisphere influenza season recommended by the World Health Organisation on September 17–19, 2008 was:

- an A/Brisbane/59/2007 (H1N1)-like virus;
- an A/Brisbane/10/2007 (H3N2)-like virus;
- a B/Florida/4/2006-like virus.

2009-2010 Northern Hemisphere Winter Season

The composition of virus vaccines for use in the 2009-2010 Northern Hemisphere influenza season recommended by the World Health Organisation on February 12, 2009 was:

- an A/Brisbane/59/2007 (H1N1)-like virus;
- an A/Brisbane/10/2007 (H3N2)-like virus;
- a B/Brisbane/60/2008-like virus.

Since the A/Brisbane/59/2007 (H1N1)-like virus used in the vaccine is an unrelated seasonal strain of influenza, it probably cannot create immunity to the new, non-seasonal strain of influenza A virus subtype H1N1 responsible for the 2009 swine flu outbreak.

2010 Southern Hemisphere Winter Season

- an A/California/7/2009 (H1N1)-like virus;

- an A/Perth/16/2009 (H3N2)-like virus;
- a B/Brisbane/60/2008-like virus.

The H1N1 strain used in this composition is the same strain used in the 2009 flu pandemic vaccine.

2010-2011 Northern Hemisphere Winter Season

The composition of virus vaccines for use in the 2010-2011 Northern Hemisphere influenza season recommended by the World Health Organisation on February 18, 2010 was:

- an A/California/7/2009 (H1N1)-like virus;
- an A/Perth/16/2009 (H3N2)-like virus;
- a B/Brisbane/60/2008-like virus.

The H1N1 strain used in this composition is the same strain used in the 2009 flu pandemic vaccine.

2011 Southern Hemisphere Winter Season

The composition of virus vaccines for use in the 2011 Southern Hemisphere influenza season recommended by the World Health Organisation on September 29, 2010 was:

- an A/California/7/2009 (H1N1)-like virus;
- an A/Perth/16/2009 (H3N2)-like virus;
- a B/Brisbane/60/2008-like virus.

The H1N1 strain used in this composition is the same strain used in the 2009 flu pandemic vaccine.

2011-2012 Northern Hemisphere Winter Season

The composition of virus vaccines for use in the 2011-2012 Northern Hemisphere influenza season recommended by the World Health Organisation on February 17, 2011 was:

- an A/California/7/2009 (H1N1)-like virus;
- an A/Perth/16/2009 (H3N2)-like virus;
- a B/Brisbane/60/2008-like virus.

The H1N1 strain used in this composition is the same strain used in the 2009 flu pandemic vaccine.

Flu Vaccine for Nonhumans

"Vaccination in the veterinary world pursues four goals:

(i) protection from clinical disease, (ii) protection from infection with virulent virus, (iii) protection from virus excretion, and (iv) serological differentiation of infected from vaccinated animals (so-called DIVA principle). In the field of influenza vaccination, neither commercially available nor experimentally tested vaccines have been shown so far to fulfil all of these requirements."

Horses

Horses with horse flu can run a fever, have a dry hacking cough, have a runny nose, and become depressed and reluctant to eat or drink for several days but usually recover in two to three weeks. "Vaccination schedules generally require a primary course of 2 doses, 3–6 weeks apart, followed by boosters at 6–12 month intervals. It is generally recognised that in many cases such schedules may not maintain protective levels of antibody and more frequent administration is advised in high-risk situations."

It is a common requirement at shows in the United Kingdom that horses be vaccinated against equine flu and a vaccination card must be produced; the FEI requires vaccination every six months.

Poultry

Poultry vaccines for bird flu are made on the cheap and are not filtered and purified like human vaccines to remove bits of bacteria or other viruses. They usually contain whole virus, not just hemagglutinin as in most human flu vaccines. Purification to standards needed for humans is far more expensive than the original creation of the unpurified vaccine from eggs. There is no market for veterinary vaccines that are that expensive. Another difference between human and poultry vaccines is that poultry vaccines are adjuvated with mineral oil, which induces a strong immune reaction but can cause inflammation and abscesses. "Chicken vaccinators who have accidentally jabbed themselves have developed painful swollen fingers or even lost thumbs, doctors said. Effectiveness may also be limited. Chicken vaccines are often only vaguely similar to circulating flu strains — some contain an H5N2 strain isolated in Mexico years ago. 'With a chicken, if you use a vaccine that's only 85 percent related, you'll get protection,' Dr. Cardona said. 'In humans, you can get a single point mutation, and a vaccine that's 99.99 percent related won't protect you.' And they are weaker than human vaccines. 'Chickens are smaller and you only need to protect them for six weeks, because that's how long they live till you eat them,' said Dr. John J. Treanor, a vaccine expert at the University of Rochester. Human seasonal flu vaccines contain about 45 micrograms of antigen, while an experimental A(H5N1) vaccine contains 180. Chicken vaccines may contain less than 1 microgram. 'You have to be careful about extrapolating data from poultry to humans,' warned Dr. David E. Swayne, director of the agriculture department's Southeast Poultry Research Laboratory. 'Birds are more closely related to dinosaurs.'"

Researchers, led by Nicholas Savill of the University of Edinburgh in Scotland, used mathematical models to simulate the spread of H5N1 and concluded that "at least 95 per cent of birds need to be protected to prevent the virus spreading silently. In practice, it is difficult to protect more than 90 per cent of a flock; protection levels achieved by a vaccine are usually much lower than this." The Food and Agriculture Organisation of the United Nations has issued recommendations on the prevention and control of avian influenza in poultry, including the use of vaccination.

A filtered and purified Influenza A vaccine for humans is being developed and many countries have recommended it be stockpiled so if an Avian influenza pandemic starts jumping to humans, the vaccine can quickly be administered to avoid loss of life. Avian influenza is sometimes called avian flu, and commonly bird flu.

Pigs

Swine origin influenza virus (SoIV) vaccines are extensively used in the swine industry in Europe and North America. Most swine flu vaccine manufacturers include an H1N1 and an H3N2 SoIV strains.

Swine influenza has become a greater problem in recent decades. Evolution of the virus has resulted in inconsistent responses to traditional vaccines. Standard commercial swine origin flu vaccines are effective in controlling the problem when the virus strains match enough to have significant cross-protection and custom (autogenous) vaccines made from the specific viruses isolated are created and used in the more difficult cases. SoIV vaccine manufacture Novartis paints this picture: "A strain of swine origin influenza virus (SoIV) called H3N2, first identified in the US in 1998, has brought exasperating production losses to swine producers. Abortion storms are a common sign. Sows go off feed for two or three days and run a fever up to 106°F. Mortality in a naïve herd can run as high as 15%."

Dogs

In 2004, Influenza A virus subtype H3N8 was discovered to cause canine influenza. Because of the lack of previous exposure to this virus, dogs have no natural immunity to this virus. However a vaccine is now available.

Computer-assisted Vaccine Design

A new parametre has been defined to quantify the antigenic distance between two H3N2 influenza strains. This parametre was used to measure antigenic distance between circulating H3N2 strains and the closest vaccine component of the influenza vaccine. For the data between 1971 and 2004, the measure of antigenic distance correlated better with efficacy in humans of the H3N2 influenza A annual vaccine than did current measures of antigenic distance such as phylogenetic sequence analysis or ferret antisera inhibition assays. This measure of antigenic distance could be used to guide the design of the annual flu vaccine. The antigenic distance combined with a multiple-strain avian influenza transmission model was used to study the threat of simultaneous introduction of multiple avian influenza strains. Population at Risk (PaR) can be used to quantify the risk of a flu pandemic and to calculate the improvement that a multiple vaccine offers.

Influenza A Virus Subtype H5N1

Influenza A virus subtype H5N1, also known as "bird flu", A(H5N1) or simply H5N1, is a subtype of the influenza A virus which can cause illness in humans and many other animal species. A bird-adapted strain of H5N1, called HPAI A(H5N1) for "highly pathogenic avian influenza virus of type A of subtype H5N1", is the causative agent of H5N1 flu, commonly known as "avian influenza" or "bird flu". It is enzootic in many bird populations, especially in Southeast Asia. One strain of HPAI A(H5N1) is spreading globally after first appearing in Asia. It is epizootic (an epidemic in nonhumans) and panzootic (affecting animals of many species, especially over a wide area), killing tens of millions of birds and spurring the culling of hundreds of millions of others to stem its spread. Most references to "bird flu" and H5N1 in the popular media refer to this strain.

According to the FAO Avian Influenza Disease Emergency Situation Update, H5N1 pathogenicity is continuing to gradually rise in endemic areas but the avian influenza disease situation in farmed birds is being held in check by vaccination. Eleven outbreaks of H5N1 were reported worldwide in June 2008 in five countries (China, Egypt, Indonesia, Pakistan and Vietnam) compared to 65 outbreaks in June 2006 and 55 in June 2007. The "global HPAI situation can be said to have improved markedly in the first half of 2008 but cases of HPAI are still underestimated and underreported in many countries because of limitations in country disease surveillance systems". On December 9, 2010 the WHO announced a total of 510 human cases which resulted in the deaths of 303 people since 2003.

A filtered and purified Influenza A vaccine for humans is being developed and many countries have recommended it be stockpiled so, if an Avian influenza pandemic starts jumping to humans, the vaccine can quickly be administered to avoid loss of life. Avian influenza is sometimes called avian flu, and commonly bird flu.

Overview

HPAI A(H5N1) is considered an avian disease, although there is some evidence of limited human-to-human transmission of the virus. A risk factor for contracting the virus is handling of infected poultry, but transmission of the virus from infected birds to humans is inefficient. Still, around 60% of humans known to have been infected with the current Asian strain of HPAI A(H5N1) have died from it, and H5N1 may mutate or reassort into a strain capable of efficient human-to-human transmission. In 2003, world-renowned virologist Robert G. Webster published an article titled "The world is teetering on the edge of a pandemic that could kill a large fraction of the human population" in *American Scientist*. He called for adequate resources to fight what he sees as a major world threat to possibly billions of lives. On September 29, 2005, David Nabarro, the newly appointed Senior United Nations System Coordinator for Avian and Human Influenza, warned the world that an outbreak of avian influenza could kill anywhere between 5 million and 150 million people. Experts have identified key events (creating new clades, infecting new species, spreading to new areas) marking the progression of an avian flu virus towards becoming pandemic, and many of those key events have occurred more rapidly than expected.

Due to the high lethality and virulence of HPAI A(H5N1), its endemic presence, its increasingly large host reservoir, and its significant ongoing mutations, the H5N1 virus is the world's largest current pandemic threat and billions of dollars are being spent researching H5N1 and preparing for a potential influenza pandemic. At least 12 companies and 17 governments are developing pre-pandemic influenza vaccines in 28 different clinical trials that, if successful, could turn a deadly pandemic infection into a nondeadly one. Full-scale production of a vaccine that could prevent any illness at all from the strain would require at least three months after the virus's emergence to begin, but it is hoped that vaccine production could increase until one billion doses were produced by one year after the initial identification of the virus.

H5N1 may cause more than one influenza pandemic as it is expected to continue mutating in birds regardless of whether humans develop herd immunity to a future pandemic strain. Influenza pandemics from its genetic offspring may include influenza A virus subtypes other than H5N1. While genetic analysis of the H5N1 virus shows that influenza pandemics from its genetic offspring can easily be far more lethal than the Spanish flu pandemic, planning for a future influenza pandemic is based on what can be done and there is no higher Pandemic Severity Index level than a Category 5 pandemic which, roughly speaking, is any pandemic as bad as the Spanish flu or worse; and for which *all* intervention measures are to be used.

Signs and Symptoms

The avian influenza hemagglutinin binds alpha 2-3 sialic acid receptors, while human influenza hemagglutinins bind alpha 2-6 sialic acid receptors. This means when the H5N1 strain infects humans, it will replicate in the lower respiratory tract, and consequently will cause viral pneumonia.

There is as yet no human form of H5N1, so all humans who have caught it so far have caught avian H5N1. In general, humans who catch a humanised influenza A virus (a human flu virus of type A) usually have symptoms that include fever, cough, sore throat, muscle aches, conjunctivitis, and, in severe cases, breathing problems and pneumonia that may be fatal. The severity of the infection depends in large part on the state of the infected person's immune system and whether the victim has been exposed to the strain before (in which case they would be partially immune). No one knows if these or other symptoms will be the symptoms of a humanised H5N1 flu.

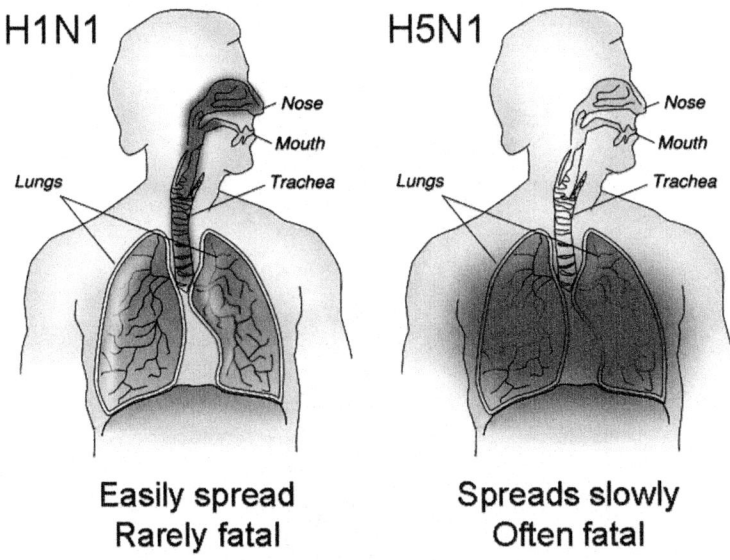

Figure : The different sites of infection of seasonal H1N1 versus avian H5N1. This influences their lethality and ability to spread.

The reported mortality rate of highly pathogenic H5N1 avian influenza in a human is high; WHO data indicate 60% of cases classified as H5N1 resulted in death. However, there is some evidence the actual mortality rate of avian flu could be much lower, as there may be many people with milder symptoms who do not seek treatment and are not counted.

In one case, a boy with H5N1 experienced diarrhea followed rapidly by a coma without developing respiratory or flu-like symptoms. There have been studies of the levels of cytokines in humans infected by the H5N1 flu virus. Of particular concern is elevated levels of tumour necrosis factor-alpha, a protein associated with tissue destruction at sites of infection and increased production of other cytokines.

Flu virus-induced increases in the level of cytokines is also associated with flu symptoms, including fever, chills, vomiting and headache. Tissue damage associated with pathogenic flu virus infection can ultimately result in death. The inflammatory cascade triggered by H5N1 has been called a 'cytokine storm' by some, because of what seems to be a positive feedback process of damage to the body resulting from immune system stimulation. H5N1 induces higher levels of cytokines than the more common flu virus types.

Genetics

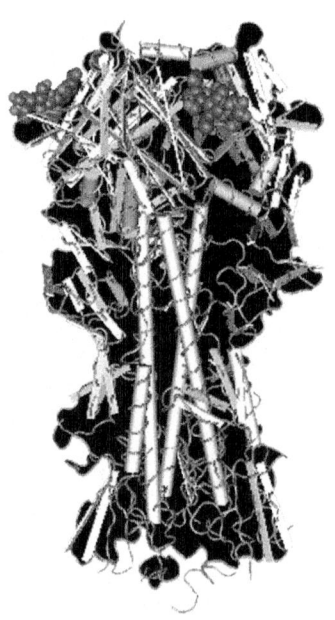

Figure : The H in H5N1 stands for "Hemagglutinin", as depicted in this molecular model

The first known strain of HPAI A(H5N1) (called A/chicken/Scotland/59) killed two flocks of chickens in Scotland in 1959; but that strain was very different from the current highly pathogenic strain of H5N1. The dominant strain of HPAI A(H5N1) in 2004 evolved from 1999 to 2002 creating the Z genotype. It has also been called "Asian lineage HPAI A(H5N1)". Asian lineage HPAI A(H5N1) is divided into two antigenic clades. "Clade 1 includes human and bird isolates from Vietnam, Thailand, and Cambodia and bird isolates from Laos and Malaysia. Clade 2 viruses were first identified in bird isolates from China, Indonesia, Japan, and South Korea before spreading westward to the Middle East, Europe, and Africa. The clade 2 viruses have been primarily responsible for human H5N1 infections that have occurred during late 2005 and 2006, according to WHO. Genetic analysis has identified six subclades of clade 2, three of which have a distinct geographic distribution and have been implicated in human infections:

- Subclade 1, Indonesia
- Subclade 2, Europe, Middle East, and Africa (called EMA)
- Subclade 3, China"

A 2007 study focused on the EMA subclade has shed further light on the EMA mutations. "The 36 new isolates reported here greatly expand the amount of whole-genome sequence data available from recent avian influenza (H5N1) isolates. Before our project, GenBank contained only 5 other complete genomes from Europe for the 2004–2006 period, and it contained no whole genomes from the Middle East or northern Africa. Our analysis showed several new findings. First, all European, Middle Eastern, and African samples fall into a clade that is distinct from other contemporary Asian clades, all of which share common ancestry with the original 1997 Hong Kong strain. Phylogenetic trees built on each of the 8 segments show a consistent picture of 3 lineages. Two of the clades contain exclusively Vietnamese isolates; the smaller of these, with 5 isolates, we label V1; the larger clade, with 9 isolates, is V2. The remaining 22 isolates all fall into a third, clearly distinct clade, labelled EMA, which comprises samples from Europe, the Middle East, and Africa. Trees for the other 7 segments display a similar topology, with clades V1, V2, and EMA clearly separated in each case. Analyses of all available complete influenza (H5N1) genomes and of 589 HA sequences placed the EMA clade as distinct from the major clades circulating in People's Republic of China, Indonesia, and Southeast Asia."

Terminology

- H5N1 isolates are identified like this actual HPAI A(H5N1) example, A/chicken/Nakorn-Patom/Thailand/CU-K2/04(H5N1):
- A stands for the species of influenza (A, B or C).
- chicken is the species the isolate was found in Nakorn-Patom/Thailand is the place this specific virus was isolated
- CU-K2 identifies it from other influenza viruses isolated at the same place 04 represents the year 2004
- H5 stands for the fifth of several known types of the protein hemagglutinin.
- N1 stands for the first of several known types of the protein neuraminidase.

Other examples include: A/duck/Hong Kong/308/78(H5N3), A/avian/NY/01(H5N2), A/chicken/Mexico/31381-3/94(H5N2), and A/shoveler/Egypt/03(H5N2). As with other avian flu viruses, H5N1 has strains called "highly pathogenic" (HP) and "low-pathogenic" (LP). Avian influenza viruses that cause HPAI are highly virulent, and mortality rates in infected flocks often approach 100%. LPAI viruses have negligible virulence, but these viruses can serve as progenitors to HPAI viruses. The current strain of H5N1 responsible for the deaths of birds across the world is an HPAI strain; all other current strains of H5N1, including a North American strain that causes no disease at all in any species, are LPAI strains. All HPAI strains identified to date have involved H5 and H7 subtypes. The distinction concerns pathogenicity in poultry, not humans. Normally a highly pathogenic avian virus is not highly pathogenic to either humans or non-poultry birds. This current deadly strain of H5N1 is unusual in being deadly to so many species, including some, like domestic cats, never previously susceptible to any influenza virus.

Genetic Structure and Related Subtypes

H5N1 is a subtype of the species *Influenza A virus* of the *Influenzavirus A* genus of the *Orthomyxoviridae* family. Like all other influenza A subtypes, the H5N1 subtype is an RNA virus. It has a segmented genome of eight negative sense, single-strands of RNA, abbreviated as PB2, PB1, PA, HA, NP, NA, MP and NS.

HA codes for hemagglutinin, an antigenic glycoprotein found on the surface of the influenza viruses and is responsible for binding the virus to the cell that is being infected. NA codes for neuraminidase, an antigenic glycosylated enzyme found on the surface of the influenza viruses. It facilitates the release of progeny viruses from infected cells. The hemagglutinin (HA) and neuraminidase (NA) RNA strands specify the structure of proteins that are most medically relevant as targets for antiviral drugs and antibodies. HA and NA are also used as the basis for the naming of the different subtypes of influenza A viruses. This is where the *H* and *N* come from in *H5N1*.

Influenza A viruses are significant for their potential for disease and death in humans and other animals. Influenza A virus subtypes that have been confirmed in humans, in order of the number of known human pandemic deaths that they have caused, include:

- H1N1, which caused the 1918 flu pandemic ("Spanish flu") and currently is causing seasonal human flu and the 2009 flu pandemic ("swine flu")
- H2N2, which caused "Asian flu"
- H3N2, which caused "Hong Kong flu" and currently causes seasonal human flu

H5N1, ("bird flu"), which is noted for having a strain (Asian-linage HPAI H5N1) that kills over half the humans it infects, infecting and killing species that were never known to suffer from influenza viruses before (e.g. cats), being unable to be stopped by culling all involved poultry - some think due to being endemic in wild birds, and causing billions of dollars to be spent in flu pandemic preparation and preventiveness

- H7N7, which has unusual zoonotic potential and killed one person
- H1N2, which is currently endemic in humans and pigs and causes seasonal human flu
- H9N2, which has infected three people
- H7N2, which has infected two people
- H7N3, which has infected two people
- H10N7, which has infected two people.

Low Pathogenic H5N1

Low pathogenic avian influenza H5N1 (LPAI H5N1) also called "North American" H5N1 commonly occurs in wild birds. In most cases, it causes minor sickness or no noticeable signs of disease in birds. It is not known to affect humans at all. The only concern about it is that it is possible for it to be transmitted to poultry and in poultry mutate into a highly pathogenic strain.

- 1975 – LPAI H5N1 was detected in a wild mallard duck and a wild blue goose in Wisconsin.
- 1981 and 1985 – LPAI H5N1 was detected in ducks by the University of Minnesota conducting a sampling procedure in which sentinel ducks were monitored in cages placed in the wild for a short period of time.
- 1983 – LPAI H5N1 was detected in ring-billed gulls in Pennsylvania.
- 1986 - LPAI H5N1 was detected in a wild mallard duck in Ohio.
- 2005 - LPAI H5N1 was detected in ducks in Manitoba, Canada.
- 2008 - LPAI H5N1 was detected in ducks in New Zealand.
- 2009 - LPAI H5N1 was detected in commercial poultry in British Columbia.

"In the past, there was no requirement for reporting or tracking LPAI H5 or H7 detections in wild birds so states and universities tested wild bird samples independently of USDA. Because of this, the above list of previous detections might not be all inclusive of past LPAI H5N1 detections. However, the World Organisation for Animal Health (OIE) recently changed its requirement of reporting detections of avian influenza. Effective in 2006, all confirmed LPAI H5 and H7 AI subtypes must be reported to the OIE because of their potential to mutate into highly pathogenic strains. Therefore, USDA now tracks these detections in wild birds, backyard flocks, commercial flocks and live bird markets."

High Mutation Rate

Influenza viruses have a relatively high mutation rate that is characteristic of RNA viruses. The segmentation of its genome facilitates genetic recombination by segment reassortment in hosts infected with two different influenza viruses at the same time. A previously uncontagious strain may then be able to pass between humans, one of several possible paths to a pandemic.

The ability of various influenza strains to show species-selectivity is largely due to variation in the hemagglutinin genes. Genetic mutations in the hemagglutinin gene that cause single amino acid substitutions can significantly alter the ability of viral hemagglutinin proteins to bind to receptors on the surface of host cells. Such mutations in avian H5N1 viruses can change virus strains from being inefficient at infecting human cells to being as efficient in causing human infections as more common human influenza virus types. This doesn't mean that one amino acid substitution can cause a pandemic, but it does mean that one amino acid substitution can cause an avian flu virus that is not pathogenic in humans to become pathogenic in humans.

Influenza A virus subtype H3N2 is endemic in pigs in China, and has been detected in pigs in Vietnam, increasing fears of the emergence of new variant strains. The dominant strain of annual flu virus in January 2006 was H3N2, which is now resistant to the standard antiviral drugs amantadine and rimantadine. The possibility of H5N1 and H3N2 exchanging genes through reassortment is a major concern. If a reassortment in H5N1 occurs, it might remain an H5N1 subtype, or it could shift subtypes, as H2N2 did when it evolved into the Hong Kong Flu strain of H3N2.

Both the H2N2 and H3N2 pandemic strains contained avian influenza virus RNA segments. "While the pandemic human influenza viruses of 1957 (H2N2) and 1968 (H3N2) clearly arose through reassortment between human and avian viruses, the influenza virus causing the 'Spanish flu' in 1918 appears to be entirely derived from an avian source".

Prevention

There are several H5N1 vaccines for several of the avian H5N1 varieties, but the continual mutation of H5N1 renders them of limited use to date: while vaccines can sometimes provide cross-protection against related flu strains, the best protection would be from a vaccine specifically produced for any future pandemic flu virus strain. Dr. Daniel Lucey, co-director of the Biohazardous Threats and Emerging Diseases graduate program at Georgetown University has made this point, "There is no H5N1 pandemic so there can be no pandemic vaccine". However, "pre-pandemic vaccines" have been created; are being refined and tested; and do have some promise both in furthering research and preparedness for the next pandemic. Vaccine manufacturing companies are being encouraged to increase capacity so that if a pandemic vaccine is needed, facilities will be available for rapid production of large amounts of a vaccine specific to a new pandemic strain.

Public Health

"The United States is collaborating closely with eight international organisations, including the World Health Organisation (WHO), the Food and Agriculture Organisation of the United Nations (FAO), the World Organisation for Animal Health (OIE), and 88 foreign governments to address the situation through planning, greater monitoring, and full transparency in reporting and investigating avian influenza occurrences. The United States and these international partners have led global efforts to encourage countries to heighten surveillance for outbreaks in poultry and significant numbers of deaths in migratory birds and to rapidly introduce containment measures. The U.S. Agency for International Development (USAID) and the U.S. Department of State, the U.S. Department of Health and Human Services (HHS), and Agriculture (USDA) are coordinating future international response measures on behalf of the White House with departments and agencies across the federal government".

Together steps are being taken to "minimise the risk of further spread in animal populations", "reduce the risk of human infections", and "further support pandemic planning and preparedness".

Ongoing detailed mutually coordinated onsite surveillance and analysis of human and animal H5N1 avian flu outbreaks are being conducted and reported by the USGS National Wildlife Health Centre, the Centres for Disease Control and Prevention, the World Health Organisation, the European Commission, and others.

Treatment

There is no highly effective treatment for H5N1 flu, but oseltamivir (commercially marketed by Roche as Tamiflu), can sometimes inhibit the influenza virus from spreading inside the user's body. This drug has become a focus for some governments and organisations trying to prepare for a possible H5N1 pandemic. On April 20, 2006, Roche AG announced that a stockpile of three million treatment courses of Tamiflu are waiting at the disposal of the World Health Organisation to be used in case of a flu pandemic; separately Roche donated two million courses to the WHO for use in developing nations that may be affected by such a pandemic but lack the ability to purchase large quantities of the drug.

However, who Expert Hassan Al-Bushra has said:

"Even now, we remain unsure about Tamiflu's real effectiveness. As for a vaccine, work cannot start on it until the emergence of a new virus, and we predict it would take six to nine months to develop it. For the moment, we cannot by any means count on a potential vaccine to prevent the spread of a contagious influenza virus, whose various precedents in the past 90 years have been highly pathogenic".

Animal and lab studies suggest that Relenza (zanamivir), which is in the same class of drugs as Tamiflu, may also be effective against H5N1. In a study performed on mice in 2000, "zanamivir was shown to be efficacious in treating avian influenza viruses H9N2, H6N1, and H5N1 transmissible to mammals". In addition, mice studies suggest the combination of zanamivir, celecoxib and mesalazine looks promising producing a 50% survival rate compared to no survival in the placebo arm. While no one knows if zanamivir will be useful or not on a yet to exist pandemic strain of H5N1, it might be useful to stockpile zanamivir as well as oseltamivir in the event of an H5N1 influenza pandemic. Neither oseltamivir nor zanamivir can currently be manufactured in quantities that would be meaningful once efficient human transmission starts. In September, 2006, a WHO scientist announced that studies had confirmed cases of H5N1 strains resistant to Tamiflu and Amantadine. Tamiflu-resistant strains have also appeared in the EU, which remain sensitive to Relenza.

Epidemiology

The earliest infections of humans by H5N1 coincided with an epizootic (an epidemic in nonhumans) of H5N1 influenza in Hong Kong's poultry population. This panzootic (a disease affecting animals of many species, especially over a wide area) outbreak was stopped by the killing of the entire domestic poultry population within the territory. However, the disease has continued to spread. On December 21, 2009 the WHO announced a total of 447 cases which resulted in the deaths of 263.

Contagiousness

H5N1 is easily transmissible between birds facilitating a potential global spread of H5N1. While H5N1 undergoes mutation and reassortment, creating variations which can infect species not previously known to carry the virus, not all of these variant forms can infect humans. H5N1 as an avian virus preferentially binds to a type of galactose receptors that populate the avian respiratory tract from the nose to the lungs and are virtually absent in humans, occurring only in and around the alveoli, structures deep in the lungs where oxygen is passed to the blood. Therefore, the virus is not easily expelled by coughing and sneezing, the usual route of transmission.

H5N1 is mainly spread by domestic poultry, both through the movements of infected birds and poultry products and through the use of infected poultry manure as fertilizer or feed. Humans with H5N1 have typically caught it from chickens, which were in turn infected by other poultry or waterfowl. Migrating waterfowl (wild ducks, geese and swans) carry H5N1, often without becoming sick. Many species of birds and mammals can be infected with HPAI A(H5N1), but the role of animals other than poultry and waterfowl as disease-spreading hosts is unknown.

According to a report by the World Health Organisation, H5N1 may be spread indirectly. The report stated that the virus may sometimes stick to surfaces or get kicked up in fertilizer dust to infect people.

Virulence

H5N1 has mutated into a variety of strains with differing pathogenic profiles, some pathogenic to one species but not others, some pathogenic to multiple species. Each specific known genetic variation is traceable to a virus isolate of a specific case of infection. Through antigenic drift, H5N1 has mutated into dozens of highly pathogenic varieties divided into genetic clades which are known from specific isolates, but all currently belonging to genotype Z of avian influenza virus H5N1, now the dominant genotype.

H5N1 isolates found in Hong Kong in 1997 and 2001 were not consistently transmitted efficiently among birds and did not cause significant disease in these animals. In 2002 new isolates of H5N1 were appearing within the bird population of Hong Kong. These new isolates caused acute disease, including severe neurological dysfunction and death in ducks.

This was the first reported case of lethal influenza virus infection in wild aquatic birds since 1961. Genotype Z emerged in 2002 through reassortment from earlier highly pathogenic genotypes of H5N1 that first infected birds in China in 1996, and first infected humans in Hong Kong in 1997. Genotype Z is endemic in birds in Southeast Asia, has created at least two clades that can infect humans, and is spreading across the globe in bird populations. Mutations are occurring within this genotype that are increasing their pathogenicity. Birds are also able to shed the virus for longer periods of time before their death, increasing the transmissibility of the virus.

Transmission and Host Range

Infected birds transmit H5N1 through their saliva, nasal secretions, feces and blood. Other animals may become infected with the virus through direct contact with these bodily fluids or through contact with surfaces contaminated with them. H5N1 remains infectious after over 30 days at 0 °C (32.0 °F) (over one month at freezing temperature) or 6 days at 37 °C (98.6 °F) (one week at human body temperature) at ordinary temperatures it lasts in the environment for weeks. In Arctic temperatures, it doesn't degrade at all.

Because migratory birds are among the carriers of the highly pathogenic H5N1 virus, it is spreading to all parts of the world. H5N1 is different from all previously known highly pathogenic avian flu viruses in its ability to be spread by animals other than poultry.

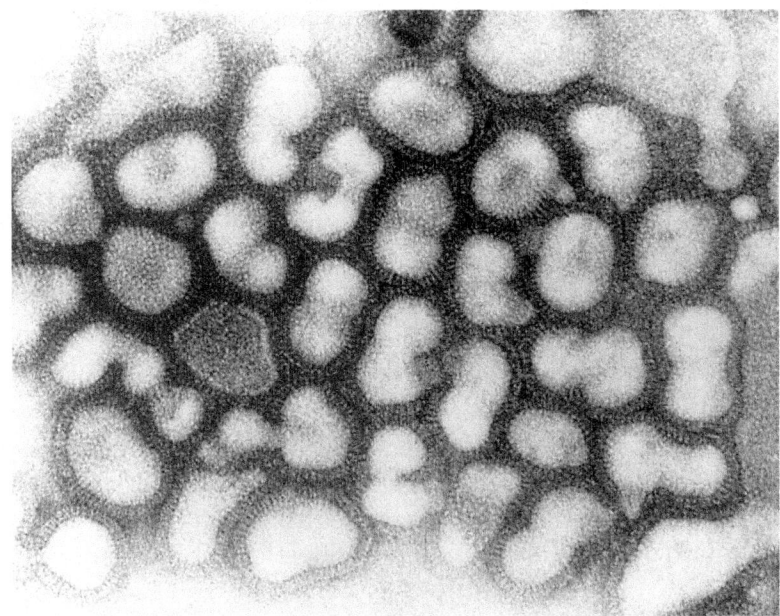

Figure : Influenza A virus, the virus that causes Avian flu. Transmission electron micrograph of negatively stained virus particles in late passage.

In October 2004, researchers discovered that H5N1 is far more dangerous than was previously believed. Waterfowl were revealed to be directly spreading the highly pathogenic strain of H5N1 to chickens, crows, pigeons, and other birds, and the virus was increasing its ability to infect mammals as well. From this point on, avian flu experts increasingly referred to containment as a strategy that can delay, but not ultimately prevent, a future avian flu pandemic.

"Since 1997, studies of influenza A (H5N1) indicate that these viruses continue to evolve, with changes in antigenicity and internal gene constellations; an expanded host range in avian species and the ability to infect felids; enhanced pathogenicity in experimentally infected mice and ferrets, in which they cause systemic infections; and increased environmental stability."

The New York Times, in an article on transmission of H5N1 through smuggled birds, reports Wade Hagemeijer of Wetlands International stating, "We believe it is spread by both bird migration and trade, but that trade, particularly illegal trade, is more important". On September 27, 2007 researchers reported that the H5N1 bird flu virus can also pass through a pregnant woman's placenta to infect the fetus. They also found evidence of what doctors had long suspected— that the virus not only affects the lungs, but also passes throughout the body into the gastrointestinal tract, the brain, liver, and blood cells.

Society and Culture

H5N1 has had a significant effect on human society, especially the financial, political, social, and personal responses to both actual and predicted deaths in birds, humans, and other animals. Billions of U.S. dollars are being raised and spent to research H5N1 and prepare for a potential avian influenza pandemic. Over ten billion dollars have been spent and over two hundred million birds killed to try to contain H5N1.

People have reacted by buying less chicken causing poultry sales and prices to fall. Many individuals have stockpiled supplies for a possible flu pandemic. International health officials and other experts have pointed out that many unknown questions still hover around the disease.

Dr. David Nabarro, Chief Avian Flu Coordinator for the United Nations, and former Chief of Crisis Response for the World Health Organisation has described himself as "quite scared" about H5N1's potential impact on humans. Nabarro has been accused of being alarmist before and on his first day in his role for the United Nations he proclaimed the avian flu could kill 150 million people. In an interview with the International Herald Tribune, Nabarro compares avian flu to AIDS in Africa, warning that underestimations led to inappropriate focus for research and intervention.

Current Status of H5N1 Candidate Vaccines

Candidate vaccines were developed in the United States and the United Kingdom during 2003 for protection against the strain that was isolated from humans in Hong Kong in February 2003 but the 2003 strain died out in 2004 making the vaccine of little use. In April 2004, WHO made an H5N1 prototype seed strain available to manufacturers. In August 2006, WHO changed the prototype strains and now offers three new prototype strains which represent three of the six subclades of the clade 2 virus which have been responsible for many of the human cases that have occurred since 2005.

The National Institute of Allergy and Infectious Diseases (NIAID) awarded H5N1 vaccine contracts to Aventis Pasteur (now Sanofi Pasteur) of Swiftwater, Pennsylvania, and to Chiron Corporation of Emeryville, California. Each manufacturer is using established techniques in which the virus is grown in eggs and then inactivated and further purified before being formulated into vaccines.

"A *universal influenza vaccine* could provide protection against all types of influenza and would eliminate the need to develop individual vaccines to specific H and N virus types. Such a vaccine would not need to be reengineered each year and could protect against an emergent pandemic strain. Developing a universal vaccine requires that researchers identify conserved regions of the influenza virus that do not exhibit antigenic variability by strain or over time. A universal vaccine is being developed by the British company Acambis and is being researched by others as well. Acambis announced in early August 2005 that it has had successful results in animal testing. The vaccine focuses on the M2 viral protein, which does not change, rather than the surface hemagglutinin and neuraminidase proteins targeted by traditional flu vaccines. The universal vaccine is made through bacterial fermentation technology, which would greatly speed up the rate of production over that possible with culture in chicken eggs, plus the vaccine could be produced constantly, since its formulation would not change. Still, such a vaccine is years away from full testing, approval, and use." As of July 2007, phase I clinical trials on humans are underway in which a vaccine that focuses on the M2 viral protein "is being administered to a small group of healthy people in order to verify the safety of the product and to provide an initial insight into the vaccine's effect on the human immune system."

In June 2006, the National Institutes of Health (NIH) began enrolling participants in a Phase 1 H5N1 study of an intranasal influenza vaccine candidate based on MedImmune's live, attenuated vaccine technology.

Oct 2010 Inovio starts a phase I clinical trial of its H5N1 vaccine (VGX-3400X).

Approved Human H5N1 Vaccines

On April 17, 2007 the US FDA approved "Influenza Virus Vaccine, H5N1" by manufacturer Sanofi Pasteur Inc for manufacture at its Swiftwater, PA facility.

In March of 2006, Hungarian Prime Minister Ferenc Gyurcsany reported that Omninvest developed a vaccine to protect humans against the H5N1 influenza strain. The vaccine was approved by the country's national pharmaceutical institute for commercial production.

Results of Trials

Early results from H5N1 clinical trials showed poor immunogenicity compared to the 15 mcg dose that induces immunity in a seasonal flu vaccine. Trials in 2006 and 2007 using two 30 mcg doses produced unacceptable results while a 2006 trial using two doses of 90 mcg each achieved acceptable levels of protection. Current flu vaccine manufacturing plants can not produce enough pandemic flu vaccine at this high dose level.

"Adjuvanted vaccines appear to hold the greatest promise for solving the grave supply-demand imbalance in pandemic influenza vaccine development. They come with obstacles—immunologic, regulatory, and commercial—but they also have generated more excitement than any other type of vaccine thus far. In August 2007, scientists working with a GlaxoSmithKline formula published a trial of a two-dose regimen of an inactivated split-virus vaccine adjuvanted with a proprietary oil-in-water emulsion; after the second injection, even the lowest dose of 3.8 mcg exceeded EU criteria for immune response. And in September, Sanofi Pasteur reported in a press release that an inactivated vaccine adjuvanted with the company's own proprietary formula induced EU-accepted levels of protection after two doses of 1.9 mcg."

The "GlaxoSmithKline-backed team that described an acceptable immune response after two adjuvanted 3.8-microgram (mcg) doses found that three fourths of their subjects were protected not only against the clade 1 Vietnam virus on which the vaccine was based, but against a drifted clade 2 virus from Indonesia as well.

To achieve prepandemic vaccines, researchers would have to ascertain the right dose and dose interval, determine how long priming lasts, and solve the puzzle of measuring primed immunity. Further, regulatory authorities would have to determine the trial design that could deliver those answers, the public discussion that would be necessary for prepandemic vaccines to be accepted, and the safety data that would need to be gathered once the vaccines went into use".

Individual Studies

Revaccination - January 2006

The purpose of this study is to determine whether having received an H5 vaccine in the past primes the immune system to respond rapidly to another dose of H5 vaccine. Subjects who participate in this study will have participated in a previous vaccine study (involving the A/Hong/Kong/97 virus) during the fall of 1998 at the University of Rochester.

A/H5N1 in Adult - February 2006

The purpose of this study is to determine the dose-related safety of flu vaccine in healthy adults. To determine the dose-related effectiveness of flu vaccine in healthy adults approximately 1 month following receipt of 2 doses of vaccine. To provide information for the selection of the best dose levels for further studies.

H5 Booster after Two doses - June 2006

The purpose of this study is to determine whether a third dose of vaccines containing A/Vietnam/1203/04 provides more immunity than two doses. Subjects who participate in this study, will have participated in DMID protocol 04-063 involving the A/Vietnam/1203/04. In this study, each subject will be asked to receive a third dose of the H5 vaccine at the same level administered in protocol 04-063.

H5 in the Elderly - August 2006

This study is intended to examine the safety and dose-related immunogenicity of three dosage levels of the Influenza A/H5N1 vaccine, as compared to saline placebo, given intramuscularly to healthy elderly adults approximately 4 weeks apart.

H5 in Healthy Adults - November 2006

This randomised, controlled, double-blinded, dose-ranging, Phase I-II study in 600 healthy adults, 18 to 49 years old, is designed to investigate the safety, reactogenicity, and dose-related immunogenicity of an investigational inactivated influenza A/H5N1 virus vaccine when given alone or combined with aluminum hydroxide. A secondary goal is to guide selection of vaccine dosage levels for expanded Phase II trials based on reactogenicity and immunogenicity profiles. This dose optimisation will be applied to both younger and older subject populations in subsequent studies. Subjects who meet the entry criteria for the study will be enrolled at one of up to 5 study sites and will be randomised into 8 groups to receive two doses of influenza A/H5N1 vaccine containing 3.75, 7.5, 15, or 45 mcg of HA with or without aluminum hydroxide adjuvant by IM injection (N= 60 or 120/vaccine dose group).

Bird flu - November 2006

This study is designed to gather critical information on the safety, tolerability, and the immunogenicity (capability of inducing an immune response) of A/H5N1 virus vaccine in healthy adults. Up to 280 healthy adults, aged 18 to 64, will participate in the study. Each subject will participate for 7 months and will be randomly placed in one of several different study groups receiving a different dose of vaccine, vaccine plus adjuvant, or placebo. All subjects will receive two injections of their assigned study product, about 28 days apart, in their muscle tissue. Subjects will keep a journal of their temperature and any adverse effects between study visits. A small amount of blood will also be drawn before the first injection, 7 days after each injection, and 6 months after the second injection.

Pandemic Flu - January 2007

This Australian study will test the safety and immunogenicity of an H5N1 pandemic influenza vaccine in healthy adults.

Children - February 2007

This is a randomised, double-blinded, placebo-controlled, staged, dose-ranging, Phase I/II study to evaluate the safety, reactogenicity, and immunogenicity of 2 doses of an IM inactivated influenza A/H5N1 vaccine in healthy children, aged 2 through 9 years. This study is designed to investigate the safety, tolerability, and dose-related immunogenicity of an investigational inactivated influenza A/H5N1 vaccine. A secondary goal is to identify an optimal dosage level of the vaccine that generates an acceptable immunogenic response, while maintaining an adequate safety profile.

Chapter 2

Broiler Management

A broiler is a type of chicken raised specifically for meat production. Modern commercial broilers, typically known as Cornish crosses or Cornish-Rocks are specially bred for large scale, efficient meat production and grow much faster than egg or traditional dual purpose breeds. They are noted for having very fast growth rates, a high feed conversion ratio, and low levels of activity. Broilers often reach a harvest weight of 4-5 pounds dressed in only five weeks.

They have white feathers and yellowish skin. This cross is also favourable for meat production because it lacks the typical "hair" which many breeds have that necessitates singeing after plucking. Both male and female broilers are slaughtered for their meat. In 2003, approximately 42 billion broilers were produced, 80% of which were produced by four companies: Aviagen, Cobb-Vantress, Hubbard Farms, and Hybro.

History

Before the development of modern commercial meat breeds (cows, chickens, etc.) broilers consisted mostly of young male chickens (cockerels) which were culled from farm flocks. The males were slaughtered for meat and the females (pullets) were kept for egg production. Compared to today, this made chicken meat scarce and expensive compared to eggs, and chicken was a luxury meat. The development of special broiler breeds decoupled the supply of broilers from the demand for eggs. This, along with advances in nutrition and incubation that allowed broilers to be raised year-round, allowed chicken to become a low-cost meat.

Broilers are often called "Rock-Cornish," referring to the adoption of a hybrid variety of chicken produced from a cross of male of a naturally double breasted Cornish strain and a female of a tall, large boned strain of white Plymouth Rocks. This first attempt at a hybrid meat breed was introduced in the 1930s and became dominant in the 1960s. The original cross was plagued by problems of low fertility, slow growth, and disease susceptibility, and modern broilers have gradually become very different from the Cornish x Rock hybrid.

Modern Variants

Access to a special diet of high protein feed delivered via an automated feeding system. This is combined with artificial lighting conditions to stimulate growth and thus the desired body weight is achieved in 4 - 8 weeks, depending on the approximate body weight required by the processing plant. After processing, the poultry is delivered as fresh or frozen chicken to the stores and supermarkets.

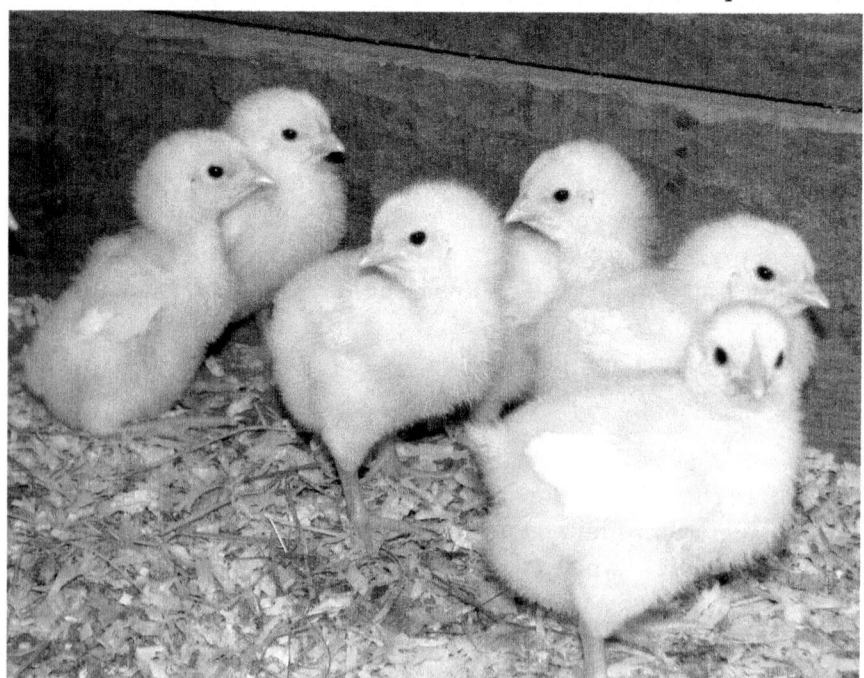

Figure : Five day old broiler strain Cornish-Rock chicks.

Because of their efficient meat conversion, broiler chickens are also popular in small family farms in rural communities, where a family will raise a small flock of broilers.

Broilers are sometimes reared on a grass range using a method called pastured poultry, as developed by Joel Salatin and promoted by the American Pastured Poultry Producers Association.

The term "broiler" is widely known in North America, Australia and England but not elsewhere in the English speaking world. The term "broiler chicken" is very widely used in Pakistan and India, as it was in the former German Democratic Republic and still nowadays in some eastern parts of Germany. The term is also used in Bangladesh, Indonesia, Sweden, Nigeria, Finland, Poland, Turkey and the Balkans.

Broiler Health Issues

Broiler chickens may develop several health issues as a result of selective breeding. Broiler chickens are bred to be very large to produce the most meat per animal. The large chickens cannot stand because their bodies grow too quickly for their legs. Therefore, they may become lame or suffer from broken legs. Broiler chickens are also prone to heart attacks for the same reason, as the heart cannot support blood flow to the large body of the chicken. Another issue with selective breeding is the larger chickens have a more aggressive appetite. The broilers are feed restricted and this leads to behavioural issues in chronically hungry birds.

Broiler chickens may often get joint disorders because their legs cannot bear the heavy bodies. A Swedish study by SLU Skara (Swedish farming university) revealed that only 1/3 of studied broiler chickens that were about to be slaughtered were healthy. Additionally, it is very inactive and as a result is a poor forager, prone to predation, and is generally not suited to small free range homestead flocks.

If the litter in the pen is not properly managed to prevent birds from standing and resting in their feces, painful hock burns and foot ulcerations and blisters can occur. Pastured birds which are rotated frequently typically do not have these issues.

Hatchery

Poultry Hatcheries

Poultry hatcheries produce a majority of the birds consumed in the developed world including chickens, turkeys, ducks and some other minor bird species. It is a multibillion dollar industry, with highly regimented production systems used to maximise bird size versus feed consumed. Birds are produced and maintained under high density, which makes production and harvesting more economical, but can also generate problems such as the spread of pathogens, which can move very quickly through the population when animal densities are high. Poultry generally start with naturally (chickens) or artificially (turkeys) inseminated hens that lay eggs; the eggs are cleaned and shells are checked for soundness before putting them in the incubators. The incubators control temperature and humidity, and turn the eggs until they hatch. Generally large numbers are produced at one time so the resulting birds are uniform in size and can be harvested at the same time. Once the eggs hatch and the chicks are a few days old, they are often vaccinated, beak-trimmed and or toe-clipped; this involves the removal of half of the top beak and the clipping of the toe ends. This is done to prevent the birds from harming each other while they are living in close proximity to each other. After these procedures, they are moved to enclosed buildings to be raised until harvest.

For chickens bred as (egg) layers, only the female chicks are considered to be of value; in excess of 100,000 male chicks can be dropped into an industrial "grinder" and disposed of in a single day.

Bantam (Poultry)

A bantam is a small variety of poultry, especially chickens. Etymologically, the name *bantam* is derived from the city of Bantam - currently known as "Banten Province" or previously "Banten Residency" - once a major seaport, in Indonesia. European sailors restocking on live fowl for sea journeys found the small native breeds of chicken in Southeast Asia to be useful, and any such small poultry came to be known as a *bantam*.

Most large chicken breeds have a bantam counterpart, sometimes referred to as a *miniature*. Miniatures are usually one-fifth to one-quarter the size of the standard breed, but they are expected to exhibit all of the standard breed's characteristics.

Characteristics

Bantams are suitable for smaller backyards as they do not need as much space as other breeds. Bantam hens are also used as laying hens, although Bantam eggs are only about one-half to one-third the size of a regular hen egg. The Bantam chicken eats the same foods as a normal chicken, chickens in the wild eat more insects and vegetation than grains. In commercial situations they are fed grain based foods because this is convenient and efficient for the producer. Bantams have become increasingly popular as pets as well as for show purposes because they are smaller and have more varied and exotic colours and feather patterns than other chickens. Breeds such as the Sebright, Dutch, and Pekin are particularly popular show birds, and true bantams.

In contrast, the Bantam rooster is famous in rural areas throughout the United Kingdom and the United States for its aggressive, "puffed-up" disposition that can be comedic in stature. It is often called a "Banty" in the rural United States.

Many bantam hens are renowned for hatching and brooding purpose. They are very protective mothers and will attack anything that gets near their young.

The Bantam chicken is considered faster and "spunkier" than their larger counterparts. In 1954, the Trinity College basketball team had named their team after the Bantam chicken. To this day, Trinity College still calls their basketball team the "Trinity Bantams".

Old English bantam roosters were commonly used for fighting in Europe. They were smaller and faster than normal roosters that were used previously.

Bantams do have a higher mortality rate when they are kept as backyard pets. They are easy targets for hawks, cats, foxes, or any other small predator. The average backyard free range bantam lives 1-3 years.

True Bantams

- A true bantam has no large counterpart, and is naturally small. Such birds are often popular for show purposes.
- Birds designated as true bantams include:
- Belgian Bearded d'Anvers
- Belgian Rumpless d'Anvers
- Belgian Bearded d'Uccle
- Belgian Rumpless d'Uccle
- Belgian Bearded de Watermael
- Booted
- Dutch
- Japanese
- Nankin

- Pekin
- Rosecomb
- Sebright
- Tuzo

Chickens, turkeys, ducks, and geese are of primary importance, while guinea fowl and squabs are chiefly of local interest.

Chickens

Humans first domesticated chickens of Indian origin for the purpose of cockfighting in Asia, Africa, and Europe. Very little formal attention was given to egg or meat production. Cockfighting was outlawed in England in 1849 and in most other countries thereafter. Exotic breeds and new standard breeds of chickens proliferated in the years to follow, and poultry shows became very popular. From 1890 to 1920 chicken raisers stressed egg and meat production, and commercial hatcheries became important after 1920.

Breeds

The breeds of chickens are generally classified as American, Mediterranean, English, and Asiatic. The American breeds of importance today are the Plymouth Rock, the Wyandotte, the Rhode Island Red, and the New Hampshire. The Barred Plymouth Rock, developed in 1865 by crossing the Dominique with the Black Cochin, has grayish-white plumage crossed with dark bars. It has good size and meat quality and is a good layer. The White Plymouth Rock, a variety of the Barred Plymouth Rock, has white plumage and is raised for its meat. Both varieties lay brown eggs. The Wyandotte, developed in 1870 from five or more strains and breeds, has eight varieties and is characterised by a plump body, excellent meat, and good egg production. Only the white strain is of any significance today because it is used in broiler crosses where its white plumage, quality of flesh, and rapid growth are highly desirable.

An American breed, the Rhode Island Red, developed in 1857 from Red Malay game fowl crossed with reddish-coloured Shanghais—with some brown Leghorn, Cornish, Wyandotte, and Brahma blood—is good for meat production and is one of the top meat breeds for the production of eggs. It has brilliant red feathers and lays brown eggs.

The New Hampshire, developed in the U.S. in 1930 from Rhode Island Red stock, is a meaty, early maturing breed with light-red feathers and lays large brown eggs. The only Mediterranean breed of importance today is the Leghorn. This breed, originated in Italy, has 12 varieties, the single-comb White Leghorn being more popular than all of the other types combined. This breed, the leading egg producer of the world, lays white eggs and is kept in large numbers in England, Canada, Australia, and the U.S. The White Minorca, a second Mediterranean breed, is often used in crossbreeding for egg production.

The only English breed of modern significance is the Cornish, a compact and heavily meated bird used in crossbreeding programs for broiler production. It is a poor producer of eggs, however.

The only Asiatic breed of significance today, the Brahma, which originated in India, has three varieties, the light Brahma being preferred because of its size.

Chicken breeding is an outstanding example of the application of basic genetic principles of inbreeding, linebreeding, and crossbreeding, as well as of intensive mass selection to effect faster and cheaper gains in broilers and maximum egg production for the egg-laying strains. Maximum use of heterosis, or hybrid vigour, through incrosses and crossbreeding has been made. Crossbreeding for egg production has used the single-comb White Leghorn, the Rhode Island Red, the New Hampshire, the Barred Plymouth Rock, the White Plymouth Rock, the Black Australorp, and the White Minorca. Crossbreeding for broiler production has used the White Plymouth Rock or New Hampshire crossed with White or Silver Cornish or incrosses utilising widely diverse inbred strains within a single breed. Rapid and efficient weight gains, and high quality, plump, meaty carcasses have been achieved thereby.

The male sperm lives in the hen's oviduct for two to three weeks. Eggs are fertilised within 24 hours after mating. Yolks originate in the ovary and grow to about 1.6 inches (4.0 centimetres) in diametre, after which they are released into the oviduct, where the thick white and two shell membranes are added. The egg then moves into the uterus where the thin white and the shell are added. This process requires a total of 24 hours per egg. The hatching of fertilised eggs requires 21 days, with the heavy breeds requiring a few more hours and the lighter breeds slightly fewer. Ideal hatching temperature approximates 100° F (38° C) with control of air flow, humidity, oxygen, and carbon dioxide being essential. Standardised egg-laying tests and official random sample tests have been used for many years to measure actual productivity.

Feeding

Chicken feeding is a highly perfected science that ensures a maximum intake of energy for growth and fat production. High quality and well-balanced protein sources produce a maximum amount of muscle, organ, skin, and feather growth.

The essential minerals produce bones and eggs; 3 to 4 percent of the live bird being composed of minerals and 10 percent of the egg. Calcium, phosphorus, sodium, chlorine, potassium, sulfur, manganese, iron, copper, cobalt, magnesium, and zinc are all required. Vitamins A, C, D, E and K and all 12 of the B vitamins are also required. Water is essential, and antibiotics are almost universally used to stimulate appetite, control harmful bacteria, and prevent disease. Modern rations produce a pound of broiler on about two pounds (0.9 kilograms) of feed and a dozen eggs from 412 pounds (2.0 kilograms) of feed.

Management

Among the world's agricultural industries, meat chicken breeding in the U.S. is one of the most advanced. It is presently considered the model for other animal industries, the broiler industry leading the way in advanced agricultural technology and efficiency. Intensive nutritional research and application, highly improved breeding stock, intelligent management, and scientific disease control have gone into the effort to give a modern broiler of uniformly high quality produced at ever-lower cost.

Today, one person can care for 25,000 to 50,000 broilers that reach market weight in three months' time, giving an annual output of from 100,000 to 200,000 broilers. A modern broiler chick gains over 43 times its initial weight in an eight-week period. Aggressive marketing methods increased the per capita consumption of broilers more than fivefold in the three decades beginning in 1950, with further substantial increases predicted for the future.

Less than half as much feed is now required to produce a pound of broiler meat as was needed in 1940. While per capita consumption of eggs has declined, the feed requirement per dozen eggs is only slightly more than half as high as it was in the early 1900s. Annual egg production per hen has increased from 104 to 244 since 1910.

A carefully controlled environment that avoids crowding, chilling, overheating, or frightening is almost universal in chicken raising. Cannibalism, which expresses itself as toe picking, feather picking, and tail picking, is controlled by debeaking at one day of age and by other management practices. The feeding, watering, egg gathering, and cleaning operations are highly mechanised. More than 90 percent of the 4,200,000,000 chicks hatched per year in the early 1980s were The vast majority of chicks hatched each year are used for broiler production and the remainder for egg production. In egg production feed represents more than two-thirds of the cost. Pullet (immature hen) flocks predominate. Hens are usually housed in wire cages with two or three hens per cage and three or four tiers of cages superposed to save space. Cages for laying hens have been found to increase production, lower mortality, reduce cannibalism, lower feeding requirements, reduce diseases and parasites, improve culling, and reduce both space and labour requirements.

Other Poultry

- These include turkeys, ducks, geese, guinea fowl, and squabs.
- Turkey production.

After World War II turkey production became highly specialised, with larger flocks predominating. Turkeys are raised in great numbers in Canada where their ancestors still live wild, as also in some parts of the U.S. Broad Breasted Bronze, Broad Breasted White, and White Holland are the most popular of the larger breeds, representing nearly three-fourths of the total production. The Beltsville Small White is the most popular of the smaller breeds and composes the bulk of the remaining 25 percent. At 24 weeks of age the toms are 50 percent heavier than the hens. In breeding flocks, one tom is required per eight or 10 hens.

Tremendous improvements both in breeding and nutrition have been made in this century. Since 1910, the amount of feed required to produce a pound of turkey meat has fallen 40 percent, while the time required has been reduced 25 percent. Fifty to 80 pounds (23–36 kilograms) of feed will produce a turkey for market weight with from 212 to 3 pounds required per pound of gain on full-size turkeys, and 212 to 234 pounds (1.1–1.2 kilograms) of feed per pound (0.45 kilograms) of gain for turkey broilers, which are marketed at from 12 to 15 weeks of age. Turkey poults are hard to start on feed. One method is to dip their beaks in water and then in feed. Another is to light the feed troughs very brightly and to use oatmeal or ground yellow corn sprinkled on top of the feed. Turkeys are given range, or open land, and automatic waterers, self-feeders, range shelters, heavy fencing, and rotated pastures are used. Successful marketing techniques have increased turkey consumption; *e.g.*, in the U.S., per capita consumption from 1930/34 to 1980 rose 500 percent.

Duck and Goose Production

Duck raising is practised on a limited scale in nearly all countries, for the most part as a small-farm enterprise. The flocks once kept in England are much reduced, the demand for eggs being greatly lessened, though a limited market still exists. Khaki Campbell and Indian Runner ducks are prolific layers, each averaging 300 eggs per year. In Indonesia, where the labour supply is large, duck herders take a flock of ducks to the high country during the warmer seasons and work their way down the mountainsides to the lowlands.

Ducks are easily transported, can be raised in close confinement, and convert some waste products and scattered grain (*e.g.*, by gleaning rice fields) to nutritious and very desirable eggs and meat. In developed countries, commercial plants have been built exclusively for duck meat production; an example is the large duckling industry of Long Island, New York. There are also local industries in The Netherlands and England, the favourite breed in England being the Aylesbury. This breed has white flesh and can reach eight pounds (3.6 kilograms) in eight weeks. The U.S. favourite is the Pekin duck, which is slightly smaller than the Aylesbury and yellow-fleshed.

Goose raising is a minor farm enterprise in practically all countries, but in Germany, Austria, some eastern European countries (notably Poland), parts of France, and locally elsewhere, there is important commercial goose production. The two outstanding meat breeds are the Toulouse, predominantly gray in colour, and the Embden (or Emden), which is white. Geese do not appear to have attracted the attention of geneticists on the same scale as the meat chicken and the turkey, and no change in the goose industry comparable to that in the others has occurred or seems to be in prospect. In some commercial plants, geese are fattened by a special process resulting in a considerable enlargement of their livers, which are sold as a delicacy, pâté de foie gras.

Guinea Fowl and Squabs

Guinea fowl are raised as a sideline on a few farms in many countries, and eaten as gourmet items. In Italy there is a fairly extensive industry.

There the birds are raised in yards with open-fronted shelters. In England, guinea fowl are marketed at 16–18 weeks of age and in the U.S. at about 10–12 weeks. The market weight is usually about 212–312 pounds, but food conversion is poor.

Pigeons are raised not only as messengers and for sport but also for the meat of their squabs (nestlings), also a gourmet item. Squab production, carried on locally, is rare in most countries with established poultry industries.

Poultry Diseases

Poultry are quite susceptible to a number of diseases; some of the more common are fowl typhoid, pullorum, fowl cholera, chronic respiratory disease, infectious sinusitis, infectious coryza, avian infectious hepatitis, infectious synovitis, bluecomb, Newcastle disease, fowl pox, avian leukosis complex, coccidiosis, blackhead, infectious laryngotracheitis, infectious bronchitis, and erysipelas.

Strict sanitary precautions, the intelligent use of antibiotics and vaccines, and the widespread use of cages for layers and confinement rearing for broilers have made it possible to effect satisfactory disease control.

Parasitic diseases of poultry, including hexamitiasis of turkeys, are caused by roundworms, tapeworms, lice, and mites. Again, modern methods of sanitation, prevention, and treatment provide excellent control.

Poussin (Chicken)

In Commonwealth countries, poussin is a butcher's term for a young chicken, less than 28 days old at slaughter and usually weighing 400-450 grammes but not above 750g. It is sometimes also called spring chicken, although the term spring chicken usually refers to chickens weighing 750-850g.

In the United States of America, *poussin* is an alternative name for a small-sized cross-breed chicken called Rock Cornish game hen, developed in the late 1950s, which is twice as old and twice as large as the typical British poussin.

Asil (Chicken)

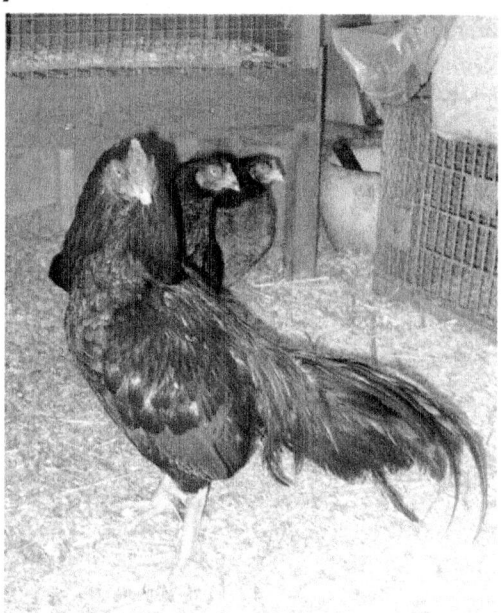

Figure : A Reza Asil cock and two hens

The Asil or Aseel is a breed of chicken originating from South Punjab/Sindh area of Pakistan and India. Similar fowl are found throughout Southeast Asia and have names like Shamo, Taiwan, etc.

Similar to Asils are Sadal (called Malay in Europe). This is a very large breed of chicken from Pakistan and India. They have longer legs with thin thighs and little wattles with pea-combs. The difference between the two is that Sadal are not game (do not fight), and Asil do. Asils were first used for cock fighting. Aseel is noted for its pugnacity. The chicks often fight when they are just a few weeks old and mature roosters will fight to the death. Hens can also be very aggressive towards each other.

Towards humans Asil are generally very tame and trusting. There are anecdotes where they have come to their keepers for other things than food, for example to get the keeper to open the door to the coop so they can get to roost.

The hens are not good layers, but are excellent sitters. Laying depends on the Asil variety, the small Asil are known to be very poor layers, sometimes laying just 6 eggs a year, whereas larger Asil can lay around 40 eggs a year.

In the U.S., the breed is listed as Critical by the American Livestock Breeds Conservancy. Aseel breed is found in almost all states of India, but abundant in Andhra Pradesh.

Breed Standard

The Asil has a distinctive upright stance, drooping tail, and well-defined musculature. Asils are good fighters The colour ranges from white to black with black breasted red being the most common.

Asil Head

The ideal Asil head is more or less round-shaped and broad, the eyes pearl white and protected by protuberant eyebrows and cheekbones, a small low set pea or walnut comb (except the single-combed Bihangham variety) with a relative short and thick beak. The colour of the face is generally red. Asil with a dark-coloured face are seen on South Indian Asil. Wattles should be absent. Only rudimentary presence is allowed.

Asil Comb Types

Asil show a variation in comb types and beak shapes. In generally we can say that North Indian Asil types such as the Reza Asil have (triple) pea combs only. The South Indian varieties such as the Malay and the Madras Asil show (triple) pea combs as well as walnut combs. Comb colour is red. Some varieties such as the Bihangham carry a single comb due to a throw back to the red jungle fowl, however these type of Asil are uncommon even in their homeland.

Wattles

Wattles should be small to absent, absent is preferred.

Asil Beak Types

The smaller the comb the better on Asil. North Indian type Asil have (triple) pea combs and a fairly large beak with the shape similar to an eagle. The birds from Southern India generally show a short but massive triangle shaped beak. Beak colour is ivory white.

Asil Eyes

Original asils have blue colour eyes when young and may turn pearl-white when grown up. Red or orange-coloured eyes are rear depending on the breed. Pale yellow-coloured eyes can be seen in young birds which lighten with age into a pearl-white colour. Sometimes pearl-white coloured eyes are seen showing tiny blood veins running in the eyes, so called "bloodshot" eyes. In some areas these are regarded as a sign of vitality.

Asil Legs

Leg colour is ivory white. Black legs are acceptable for black colour Asils. The other main leg colours within the Asil breed are pale,grey and white, black, though they are considered inferior. The dark-coloured leg colours are generally seen on the South Indian Asil. Some Asil show very rough scales pointing a little bit outwards. One the ways you recognise an asil (aseel) is by the legs if they are yellow it means there not pure aseel. what they could be is a shamo, taiwaan or other game birds.

Asil Body Description

The Asil should have broad shoulders and wings are carried against the body. The body of an Asil is very muscular but also compact.

Varieties

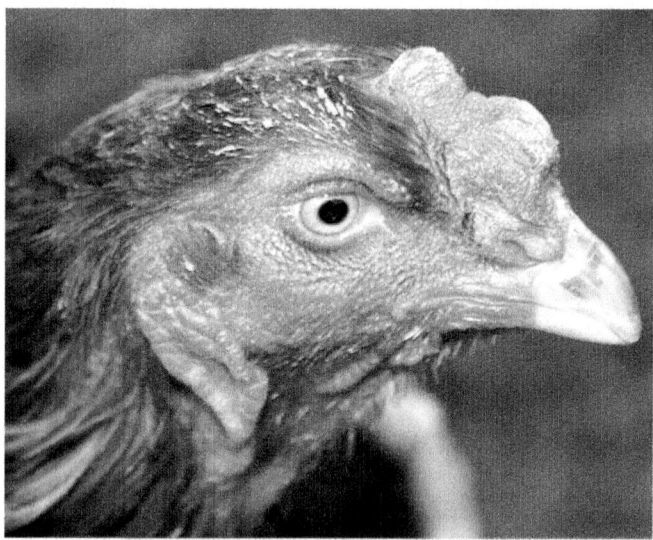

Figure : Portrait of Kulang Asil rooster head

There are many varieties of Asil, some are standardised for shows such as the Reza Asil in the UK, some are simply named after the area where they are bred such as the Mianwali Asil from Pakistan or the colour, red/wheaten Asil are generally known as "Sonatol".

There are also hen-feathered Asil knows as "Madaroo" these are found in various colours, but the cocks come with feathers in hen colour, don't have sickle feathers in the tails and miss the large hanging feathers on the saddle. This variety is very rare.

Asil with feather beards under their beaks known as "muffed" and with tufts on the top of their heads known as "tasseled" are also seen, but are very rare especially outside India/Pakistan.

Bhaingam Asil variety have a have a large single comb but confirm to all the other Asil standards.

Broadly speaking, Asil in Europe are categorised and shown under these three types: Madras asil Madras asils are very big and muscular. They can get up to 32 inches the main colours are black, red, grey, blue and green.

Reza Asil

Height: Up to 50 cms tall. Weight: Maximum weight for the hens is 1.8 kg, max weight for the cocks is 2.7 kg.

This type is standardised by the Asian Hardfeather Society in the UK and is seen at shows throughout the UK, but is quite rare.

This group of Asil reached worldwide popularity due to books and articles written by gamefowl experts such as Herbert Atkinson, Siran and Paul Deraniyagala from Sri Lanka and Carlos Finsterbusch from Chile. The Reza Asil family according the old (Western) gamefowl literature is subdivided into following strains: (Amir) Ghan (Dark-Red), Sonatol(Light-Red), (Siyah) Rampur(Black), Kalkatiya (Kaptan)(Speckled-Reds) and Jawa(Duckwing). All these strains are identified by their specific colour, these colours do not necessarily correspond with the area where the birds come from.

In colonial times other colours such as whites, spangles, golden etc. were regarded as inferior. At present day the "classic" strains and names given mentioned by Atkinson are more or less forgotten. The native people in India, Pakistan, Bangladesh and Sri Lanka only know the Reza-type Asil by their local names.

Kulang Asil

Height: Up to 75 cms Tall. Weight: 5 to 7 kg.

The large Asil are divided into sub-varieties : North Indian, South Indian and Madras type. The North and South Indian varieties don't differ much. Only type of comb, shape of the beak and body shape are different. For example : Northern type = slender, Southern type = heavier build. The Madras Asil however is significantly different. They have a lower station, are heavier build and stronger boned. These birds often come in a bluish colour. This variety is found in the deep south of India, the Tamil Nadu state.

Sindhi Breed

It is one of the tallest and biggest breed of Asils. Main colours are red and blue. They are mostly fought in the Sindh area of Pakistan. These aseels have good endurance and usually their fights last longer than Mianwali Aseels. With the arrival of Mianwali they have started to disappear from the fights.

Mianwali Breed

This breed is mainly found in Mianwali district of Pakistan. However since its arrival, this breed has risen to popularity in Pakistan, currently the primary game breed used in the pits also preferred by gamblers. It is smaller compared to Sindhi aseels weighing between 1.5 to 3.5 kg depending on the preference of breeders. It is much faster and a better head hitter usually comes in small to medium height. A good Mianwali aseel should kill its opponent with in few minutes. They have been known to kill bigger roosters because of their speed and accuracy. They come in various colours such as Java (duckwing), Lakha (reddish), black and various others depending on the combination used in breeding. Very hard and a brave fighter with attitude to inspire, excellent in naked heels and metal spurs. There are many sub breeds of this breed owing to the combination used in breeding. A good tested Mianwali rooster would usually have offspring of a similar quality. Typical description would be small curved beak, strong joints, pearl/white/yellow eye colour, short crow, small comb and do not have heavy body structure. May look smaller than other breeds but is excellent spurer.

Amroha

This is a rare breed of Aseel used in Pakistan and India. Very few of these roosters exist in their pure form. They are known to be small to medium like Mianwali. It is also known that they are champion of naked heel fighting. In simple, it is a fantasy of most aseel breeders in Pakistan.

Bantam Asil

Weight: Up to 0.75 kg.

Bantam Asil have been created at the end of the 19th century by an English breeder named William Flamank Entwisle. The breed got very popular after its creation but after a couple of decades interest in this variety slowly died out.

Until the beginning of the 1980s nothing was heard about these little Asil. A Belgian breeder named Willy Coppens created them again using Shamo (chicken), Indian Game and Reza Asil. The breed was also introduced again in Holland and United Kingdom. At present day Bantam Asil are quite popular and they are bred in various colours.

Brahma (Chicken)

Brahmas are an Asiatic breed of chicken, originating in the Brahmaputra region in India where they were known as "Gray Chittagongs." Their heritage is unclear, but they are believed to be closely related to the Jungle Fowl (Gallus Gigantus) and the Cochin. The first Brahmas were brought to the U.S. from British India in 1846, and were used as a utility fowl for their edibility and generous egg laying and hardiness even during the winter months, although today they are kept mainly for ornamental purposes as selection for utility has taken a back seat to selection for appearance.

Some of the earliest imports to the U.S. reached weights of nearly 14 pounds, but rarely is such massive size seen today: standard weight for a cock is 11 pounds; hens are 8.5 pounds. By the 1870s Brahmas had become so popular that they were admitted into the American Poultry Association's Standard of Perfection.

Temperament

Brahmas are calm, friendly birds that make good pets or exhibition fowl. Males are calm and generally not aggressive towards humans. They are not skittish or easily scared, making them a popular choice for families with children.

Due to their docile demeanour, Brahmas can be easily trained so that they can be handled by almost anyone. They should be hand trained when young because their large size makes them difficult to control in the early stages of training if they are full grown.

Appearance

Brahmas are massive in appearance, in part due to profuse, loose feathering and feathered legs and toes. Approximate weights:

Cock - 12 pounds (5.443 kg)

Cockerel - 10 pounds (4.536 kg)

Hen - 9 pounds

Pullet - 8 pounds

Recognised Varieties

The American Standard of Perfection recognises three Brahma varieties: light, dark, and buff. The light Brahma has a base colour of white, with black hackles edged in white and a black tail. The cocks' saddle feathers in a light Brahma are striped with black. The dark Brahma has the most notable difference between cock and hen. The hen has a dark gray and black pencilled coloration with the same hackle as the light whereas the cock has black and white hackles and saddle feathers, and a black base and tail. The wings of a dark Brahma are white-shouldered and the primary feathers (remiges) are edged with white. Buff Brahmas have the same pattern of black as light Brahmas, except with a golden buff base colour instead of white. In Australia Brahma Breeders are creating more colours and along with the accepted American varieties - Light, dark, and buff the Australian Poultry Association have accepted black, blue, partridge, crele and even barred varieties of Brahma.

Intensive Chicken Farming

In egg-producing farms, birds are typically housed in rows of battery cages. Environmental conditions are automatically controlled, including light duration, which mimics summer daylength. This stimulates the birds to continue to lay eggs all year round. Normally, significant egg production only occurs in the warmer months. Critics argue that year-round egg production stresses the birds more than normal seasonal production.

Meat chickens, commonly called broilers, are floor-raised on litter such as wood shavings or rice hulls, indoors in climate-controlled housing. Poultry producers routinely use nationally approved medications, such as antibiotics, in feed or drinking water, to treat disease or to prevent disease outbreaks arising from overcrowded or unsanitary conditions. In the U.S., the national organisation overseeing chicken production is the Food and Drug Administration (F.D.A.). Some F.D.A.-approved medications are also approved for improved feed utilisation. In the U.S., federal law prohibits the use of hormones or steroids in poultry production.

In egg-producing farms, cages allow for more birds per unit area, and this allows for greater productivity and lower space and food costs, with more efforts put into egg-laying. In the U.S., for example, the current recommendation by the United Egg Producers is 67 to 86 in^2 (430 to 560 cm^2) per bird, which is about 9 inches by 9 inches. Modern poultry farming is very efficient and allows meat and eggs to be available to the consumer in all seasons at a lower cost than free range production, and the poultry have no exposure to predators.

The cage environment of egg producing does not permit birds to roam. The closeness of chickens to one another frequently causes cannibalism. Cannibalism is controlled by debeaking (removing a portion of the bird's beak with a hot blade so the bird cannot effectively peck). Another condition that can occur in prolific egg laying breeds is osteoporosis. This is caused from year-round rather than seasonal egg production, and results in chickens whose legs cannot support them and so can no longer walk. During egg production, large amounts of calcium are transferred from bones to create eggshell. Although dietary calcium levels are adequate, absorption of dietary calcium is not always sufficient, given the intensity of production, to fully replenish bone calcium.

Under intensive farming methods, a meat chicken will live less than six weeks before slaughter. This is half the time it would take traditionally. This compares with free-range chickens which will usually be slaughtered at 8 weeks, and organic ones at around 12 weeks.

In intensive broiler sheds, the air can become highly polluted with ammonia from the droppings. This can damage the chickens' eyes and respiratory systems and can cause painful burns on their legs (called hock burns) and feet. Chickens bred for fast growth have a high rate of leg deformities because they cannot support their increased body weight. Because they cannot move easily, the chickens are not able to adjust their environment to avoid heat, cold or dirt as they would in natural conditions. The added weight and overcrowding also puts a strain on their hearts and lungs. In the U.K., up to 19 million chickens die in their sheds from heart failure each year.

Chapter 3

Poultry Farming in the United States

In the United States, chickens were raised primarily on family farms until about 1960. Originally, the primary value in poultry keeping was eggs, and meat was considered a by product of egg production. Its supply was less than the demand, and poultry was expensive. Except in hot weather, eggs can be shipped and stored without refrigeration for some time before going bad; this was important in the days before widespread refrigeration.

Farm flocks tended to be small because the hens largely fed themselves through foraging, with some supplementation of grain, scraps, and waste products from other farm ventures. Such feedstuffs were in limited supply, especially in the winter, and this tended to regulate the size of the farm flocks. Soon after poultry keeping gained the attention of agricultural researchers (around 1896), improvements in nutrition and management made poultry keeping more profitable and businesslike.

Prior to about 1910, chicken was served primarily on special occasions or Sunday dinner. Poultry was shipped live or killed, plucked, and packed on ice (but not eviscerated). The "whole, ready-to-cook broiler" wasn't popular until the 1950s, when end-to-end refrigeration and sanitary practices gave consumers more confidence. Before this, poultry were often cleaned by the neighbourhood butcher, though cleaning poultry at home was a commonplace kitchen skill.

Two kinds of poultry were generally offered: broilers or "spring chickens," young male chickens, a by product of the egg industry, which were sold when still young and tender (generally under 3 pounds live weight); and "fowls" or "stewing hens," also a by product of the egg industry, which were old hens past their prime for laying. This is no longer practised; modern meat chickens are a different breed. Egg-type chicken carcasses no longer appear in stores.

The major milestone in 20th century poultry production was the discovery of Vitamin-D (named in 1922), which made it possible to keep chickens in confinement year-round. Before this, chickens did not thrive during the winter (due to lack of sunlight), and egg production, incubation, and meat production in the off-season were all very difficult, making poultry a seasonal and expensive proposition. Year-round production lowered costs, especially for broilers.

Improvements in production and quality were accompanied by lower labour requirements. In the 1930s through the early 1950s, 1,500 hens was considered to be a full-time job for a farm family. In the late Fifties, egg prices had fallen so dramatically that farmers typically tripled the number of hens they kept, putting three hens into what had been a single-bird cage or converting their floor-confinement houses from a single deck of roosts to triple-decker roosts. Not long after this, prices fell still further and large numbers of egg farmers left the business. This marked the beginning of the transition from family farms to larger, vertically integrated operations.

Robert Plamondon reports that the last family chicken farm in his part of Oregon, Rex Farms, had 30,000 layers and survived into the Nineties. But the standard laying house of the surviving operations is around 125,000 hens.

This fall in profitability was accompanied by a general fall in prices to the consumer, allowing poultry and eggs to lose their status as luxury foods.

The vertical integration of the egg and poultry industries was a late development, occurring after all the major technological changes had been in place for years (including the development of modern broiler rearing techniques, the adoption of the Cornish Cross broiler, the use of laying cages, etc.).

By the late 1950s, poultry production had changed dramatically. Large farms and packing plants could grow birds by the tens of thousands. Chickens could be sent to slaughterhouses for butchering and processing into prepackaged commercial products to be frozen or shipped fresh to markets or wholesalers. Meat-type chickens currently grow to market weight in six to seven weeks whereas only fifty years ago it took three times as long. This is due to genetic selection and nutritional modifications (and not the use of growth hormones, which are illegal for use in poultry in the US and many other countries).

Once a meat consumed only occasionally, the common availability and lower cost has made chicken a common meat product within developed nations. Growing concerns over the cholesterol content of red meat in the 1980s and 1990s further resulted in increased consumption of chicken.

Current Status

Today, eggs are produced on large egg ranches on which environmental parametres are controlled. Chickens are exposed to artificial light cycles to stimulate egg production year-round. In addition, it is a common practice to induce moulting through manipulation of light and the amount of food they receive in order to further increase egg size and production.

On average, a chicken lays one egg a day for a number of days (a "clutch"), then does not lay for one or more days, then lays another clutch. Originally, the hen presumably laid one clutch, became broody, and incubated the eggs. Selective breeding over the centuries has produced hens that lay more eggs than they can hatch. Some of this progress was ancient, but most occurred after 1900. In 1900, average egg production was 83 eggs per hen per year. In 2000, it was well over 300.

In the United States, laying hens are butchered after their second egg laying season. In Europe, they are generally butchered after a single season. The laying period begins when the hen is about 18–20 weeks old (depending on breed and season). Males of the egg-type breeds have little commercial value at any age, and all those not used for breeding (roughly fifty percent of all egg-type chickens) are killed soon after hatching. Such "day-old chicks" are sometimes sold as food for captive and falconers birds of prey. The old hens also have little commercial value. Thus, the main sources of poultry meat a hundred years ago (spring chickens and stewing hens) have both been entirely supplanted by meat-type broiler chickens.

Traditionally, chicken production was distributed across the entire agricultural sector. In the twentieth century, it gradually moved closer to major cities to take advantage of lower shipping costs. This had the undesirable side effect of turning the chicken manure from a valuable fertilizer that could be used profitably on local farms to an unwanted by product. This trend may be reversing itself due to higher disposal costs on the one hand and higher fertilizer prices on the other, making farm regions attractive once more. •

From the farmer's point of view, eggs used to be practically the same as currency, with general stores buying eggs for a stated price per dozen. Egg production peaks in the early spring, when farm expenses are high and income is low. On many farms, the flock was the most important source of income, though this was often not appreciated by the farmers, since the money arrived in many small payments. Eggs were a farm operation where even small children could make a valuable contribution.

Production Statistics

Eggs

Table : Total egg production in the United States

Year	Eggs produced (millions)
2007	91,101
2008	90,151
2009	90,484
2010	91,398

Individual States

Table : Egg production by state, 2010

State	Eggs produced (millions)
AL	2,182
AR	2,894
CA	5,390
CO	1,066
CT	695
FL	2,592
GA	4,419
HI	69.5
IL	1,272
IN	6,493
IA	14,614
KY	1,119
LA	462
ME	1,034

MD	616
MA	36
MI	2,912
MN	2,869
MS	1,467
MO	1,949
MT	119
NE	2,751
NY	1,161
NC	3,251
OH	7,535
OK	769
OR	715
PA	6,976
SC	1,102
SD	672
TN	308
TX	4,811
UT	929
VT	59
VA	729
WA	1,739
WV	267
WI	1,312
WY	2.4
	2,042

Meat

In 2008, 9.08 billion chickens were slaughtered in the United States according to United States Department of Agriculture data.

Recommended Culling Practices

The American Veterinary Medical Association recommends cervical dislocation and asphyxiation by carbon dioxide as the best options, but has recently amended their guidelines to include maceration, putting non-anaesthetised chicks through a grinder. The 2005-2006 American Veterinary Medical Association Executive Board held its final meeting July 13 in Honolulu, prior to the 2006 session of the House of Delegates and the AVMA Annual Convention. It proposed a policy change, which was recommended by the Animal Welfare Committee on disposal of unwanted chicks, poults, and pipped eggs.

The new policy states, in part, "Unwanted chicks, poults, and pipped eggs should be killed by an acceptable humane method, such as use of a commercially designed macerator that results in instantaneous death.

Smothering unwanted chicks or poults in bags or containers is not acceptable. Pips, unwanted chicks, or poults should be killed prior to disposal. A pipped egg, or pip, is one where the chick or poult has not been successful in escaping the egg shell during the hatching process."

Environmental Issues

The Illinois River, which flows between Arkansas and Oklahoma, has had a high level of pollution due to water runoff contaminated with chicken manure.

Why did the chicken cross the road?

"Why did the chicken cross the road?" is a common riddle or joke in several languages. The answer or punchline is: "To get to the other side". The riddle is an example of anti-humour, in that the curious setup of the joke leads the listener to expect a traditional punchline, but they are instead given a simple statement of fact. Since its inception, "Why did the chicken cross the road?" has become largely iconic as an exemplary generic joke to which most people know the answer, and has been repeated and changed numerous times.

The earliest known appearance was in 1847 in *The Knickerbocker*, a New York City monthly magazine:

There are 'quips and quillets' which seem actual conundrums, but yet are none. Of such is this: 'Why does a chicken cross the street? Are you 'out of town?' Do you 'give it up?' Well, then: 'Because it wants to get on the other side!'

The joke had become widespread by the 1890s, when a variant version appeared in the magazine *Potter's American Monthly*:

Why should not a chicken cross the road?

It would be a fowl proceeding.

Variations

There are many riddles that assume a familiarity with this well-known riddle and its answer. One class of variations enlist a creature other than the chicken to cross the road, in order to refer back to the original chicken joke. For example, a turkey or duck crosses "because it was the chicken's day off," and a dinosaur "because chickens didn't exist yet."

Punning variations include "Why didn't the skeleton cross the road?" to which possible answers may be "Because he had no guts" or "Because he had no body to go with him", and "Why did the chicken cross the road halfway? To 'lay it on the line'." Some variants are both puns and references to the original joke, such as "Why did the duck cross the road?" "To prove he's no chicken." Another variant is "Why did the chicken cross the playground?" to which the answer is "To get to the other slide."

Another class of variations, designed for written rather than oral transmission, employs parody by pretending to have notable individuals or institutions give characteristic answers to the question posed by the riddle. As with the lightbulb joke, variants on this theme are virtually endless.

Chicken Fat

Chicken fat is fat obtained (usually as a by-product) from chicken rendering and processing. Of animal-sourced substances, chicken fat is noted for being high in linoleic acid, a beneficial omega-6 fatty acid. Linoleic acid levels are between 17.9% and 22.8%. It is often used in pet foods, and has also been used in the production of biodiesel. Chicken fat is one of two types of animal fat referred to as Schmaltz, the other being goose fat.

Disease

Aspergillosis

Aspergillosis is the name given to a wide variety of diseases caused by fungi of the genus *Aspergillus*. The most common forms are allergic bronchopulmonary aspergillosis, pulmonary aspergilloma and invasive aspergillosis. Most humans inhale *Aspergillus* spores every day. Aspergillosis develops mainly in individuals who are immunocompromised, either from disease or from immunosuppressive drugs, and is a leading cause of death in acute leukemia and hematopoietic stem cell transplantation. Conversely, it may also develop as an allergic response. The most common cause is *Aspergillus fumigatus.*

Symptoms

A fungus ball in the lungs may cause no symptoms and may be discovered only with a chest X-ray, or it may cause repeated coughing up of blood and occasionally severe, even fatal, bleeding. A rapidly invasive *Aspergillus* infection in the lungs often causes cough, fever, chest pain, and difficulty breathing.

Aspergillosis affecting the deeper tissues makes a person very ill. Symptoms include fever, chills, shock, delirium, and blood clots. The person may develop kidney failure, liver failure (causing jaundice), and breathing difficulties. Death can occur quickly.

Aspergillosis of the ear canal causes itching and occasionally pain. Fluid draining overnight from the ear may leave a stain on the pillow. Aspergillosis of the sinuses causes a feeling of congestion and sometimes pain or discharge.

In addition to the symptoms, an X-ray or computerised tomography (CT) scan of the infected area provides clues for making the diagnosis. Whenever possible, a doctor sends a sample of infected material to a laboratory to confirm identification of the fungus.

Diagnosis

On chest X-ray and CT, pulmonary aspergillosis classically manifests as an air crescent sign. In hematologic patients with invasive aspergillosis, the galactomannan test can make the diagnosis in a noninvasive way.

On microscopy, *Aspergillus* species are reliably demonstrated by silver stains, e.g., Gridley stain or Gomori methenamine-silver. These give the fungal walls a gray-black colour. The hyphae of Aspergillus species range in diametre from 2.5 to 4.5 µm. They have septate hyphae, but these are not always apparent, and in such cases they may be mistaken for Zygomycota. *Aspergillus* hyphae tend to have dichotomous branching that is progressive and primarily at acute angles of about 45°.

Treatment

The current treatments include voriconazole and liposomal amphotericin B. Newer findings suggest use of mild oral steroids for a longer period of time, preferably for 6-9 months in aspergillosis in pulmonary segment.

Other drugs used, such as amphotericin B, caspofungin (in combination therapy only), flucytosine (in combination therapy only) or itraconazole, are used to treat this fungal infection. However, a growing proportion of infections are resistant to the triconazoles.

Infections in Animals

Albeit relatively rare in humans, aspergillosis is a common and dangerous infection in birds, particularly in pet parrots. Mallards and other ducks are particularly susceptible, as they will often resort to poor food sources during bad weather. Captive raptors, such as falcons and hawks, are susceptible to this disease if they are kept in poor conditions and especially if they are fed pigeons, which are often carriers of "asper".

Aspergillosis has been the culprit in several recent rapid die-offs among waterfowl. From 8 December until 14 December 2006, over 2,000 Mallards died in the Burley, Idaho area, an agricultural community approximately 150 miles southeast of Boise. Moldy waste grain from the farmland and feedlots in the area is the suspected source. A similar aspergillosis outbreak caused by mouldy grain killed 500 Mallards in Iowa in 2005.

While there is no connection between aspergillosis and the H5N1 strain of avian influenza (commonly called "bird flu"), rapid die-offs caused by aspergillosis can spark fears of bird flu outbreaks. Laboratory analysis is the only way to distinguish bird flu from aspergillosis.

Primary Cutaneous Aspergillosis

Primary cutaneous aspergillosis is a rare skin condition most often occurring at the site of intravenous cannulas in immunosuppressed patients.

Otomycosis

Otomycosis (also known as Singapore Ear) is a fungal ear infection, a superficial mycotic infection of the outer ear canal. It is more common in the tropical countries. The infection may be either subacute or acute and is characterised by inflammation, pruritus, scaling, and severe discomfort. The mycosis results in inflammation, superficial epithelial exfoliation, masses of debris containing hyphae, suppuration, and pain.

Clinical Finding

The most characteristic finding on ear examination is the presence of greyish white thick debris known as "wet blotting paper". Most fungal ear infections are caused by Aspergillus niger and Candida albicans, but exceptions exist.

Treatment

Otomycosis is treated with azole antifungals, and symptomatically managed with oral antihistamines.

Avian Sarcoma Leukosis Virus

Avian sarcoma leukosis virus (ASLV) is an endogenous retrovirus that infects and can lead to cancer in chickens; experimentally it can infect other species of birds and mammals. ASLV replicates in chicken embryo fibroblasts, the cells that contribute to the formation of connective tissues. Different forms of the disease exist, including lymphoblastic, erythroblastic, and osteopetrotic.

Avian Sarcoma Leukosis Virus is characterised by a wide range of tumours, the most common of which are lymphomas. The disease is also characterised by an enlarged liver due to infiltration of cancerous lymphoid cells. In addition, other abdominal organs and the bursa of Fabricius are often infected.

History

Sarcoma in chickens has been studied since the early 1900s when Ellerman and Bang demonstrated that erythroleukemia can be transmitted between chickens by cell-free tissue filtrates, and in 1911 when (Francis) Peyton Rous proved that sarcoma can be transmitted through cell free extracts of solid chicken tumours. Rous was awarded the Nobel Prize for his discovery in 1966.

By the 1960s, ASLV became a problem with egg-laying hens and effort was made to isolate the disease. However, the movement was unsuccessful in maintaining leukosis-free flocks. In 1961, Rous sarcoma virus (RSV), which is closely related to ASLV, was shown to contain RNA, and oncogenic viruses, such as RSV and ASLV, were termed RNA tumor viruses. By the late 1960s, Howard Temin hypothesized that RSV made a copy of its own DNA and integrated that into the host cell's chromosomal DNA. Much debate in the scientific community surrounded this issue until DNA integration was demonstrated by

Temin in 1968 and reverse transcriptase was independently discovered by both Temin and David Baltimore in 1970. Temin and Baltimore won the Nobel Prize in Medicine in 1975.

Today, research is carried out on ASLV in order to better understand retroviral cell entry. Since ASLV uses distinct cellular receptors to gain entry into cells, it has proven useful for understanding the early events in retroviral infection. A detailed understanding of retroviral cell entry may lead to the discovery of ways in which to block the viruses from entering cells. Retroviruses also have the potential to serve as gene delivery vectors in gene therapy.

Classification

ASLV is a Group VI virus of the family *Retroviridae*. It is of the *Alpharetrovirus* genus, and has a C-type morphology. Hence, it is an enveloped virus with a condensed, central core, and has barely visible envelope spikes, or proteins.

ASLV is divided into six subgroups, labelled A through E and J, each having a different antigenicity due to variances in viral envelope glycoproteins. Strains A through E are highly related and are believed to have evolved from the same ancestor. The subgroups evolved to utilise difference cellular receptors to gain entry into avian cells due to the host developing resistance to viral entry. Some antigenic variation can occur within subgroups, and all strains are oncogenic, but oncogenicity and the ability to replicate varies between subgroups.

Viral Structure and Composition

Like many retroviruses, ASLV consists of a lipid envelope containing transmembrane and cell surface glycoproteins. Enclosed within the envelope is a capsid surrounding single stranded RNA, integrase, protease, and reverse transcriptase, an enzyme that allows for the reversal of genetic transcription. As with all retroviruses, the virus is transcribed from RNA to DNA, instead of DNA to RNA as in normal cellular replication.

Viral glycoprotein-receptor interactions are required to initiate membrane fusion of the virus and cell. The surface glycoproteins contain the major domains that interact with the host cell receptor while the transmembrane (TM) glycoproteins anchor the surface glycoproteins to the virus membrane. The TM glycoproteins are directly involved in the fusion of the virus and host membranes for entry. The surface glycoproteins for subgroups A-E are almost identical and include the conservation of all cysteine amino acid residues. Viral specificity is determined by five hyper variable regions, vr1, vr2, hr1, hr2, and vr3, on the surface glycoproteins. Binding specificity is determined primarily by the hr1 and hr2 regions, with the vr3 region contributing to receptor recognition but not to binding specificity of the viral glycoprotein and cellular receptor.

In chicken chromosomes, three autosomal loci, t-va, t-vb, and t-vc, have been identified which control cell susceptibility of the ASLV virus subgroups A, B, and C respectively. Each of these genes codes for the cellular receptors Tva, Tvb, and Tvc.

Tva contains sequences related to the ligand binding region of low-density lipoprotein receptors (LDLR). The Tvb receptor is believed to be very closely related to the receptors for both ASLV D and E, so that the ASLV D and E will bind to Tvb. Tvb is a member of the tumour necrosis factor receptor (TNFR) family. The Tvc receptor is closely related to mammalian butyrophilins, which are members of the immunoglobulin superfamily.

ASLV is genetically closely related to the Rous sarcoma virus (RSV), but unlike RSV, ASLV does not contain the *src* gene, which codes for a tyrosine kinase, and does not transform the fibroblasts that it infects.

Both RSV and ASLV contain the *gag* gene, which is common to most retroviruses and encodes for the capsid proteins, and the *pol* gene which encodes for the reverse transcriptase enzyme. ASLV and some RSVs also contain the *env* gene, which encodes a precursor polyprotein that assembles in the endoplasmic reticulum. The polyproteins are then transported to the Golgi apparatus, glycosylated and cleaved to produce two glycoproteins: one surface and one transmembrane.

Avian Sarcoma Leukosis Virus

Table : Virus classification

Group:	Group VI (ssRNA-RT)
Family:	*Retroviridae*
Subfamily:	*Orthoretrovirinae*
Genus:	*Alpharetrovirus*
Species:	*Avian leucosis virus*

Blackhead Disease

Blackhead disease (also known simply as *blackhead*) is a commercially important avian disease that affects chickens, turkeys and other poultry birds. The disease carries a high mortality rate and primarily affects the liver and cecum. It is a form of histomoniasis which is transmitted by the protozoan parasite *Histomonas meleagridis*. The protozoan is in turn transmitted by the nematode parasite *Heterakis gallinarum. H. meleagridis* resides within the eggs of *H. gallinarum* so that birds ingest the parasites along contaminated soil or food. Earthworms can act as a paratenic host. Symptom of the infection is characterised by the development of cyanotic (bluish) discoloration on the head and hence the common name, but apparently a misnomer, of the disease, "blackhead".

Poultry (especially free-ranging) and wild birds, commonly harbour a number of parasitic worms with only mild health problems for them. Turkeys are much more susceptible to getting blackhead than are chicken. Thus chicken can be infected carriers for a long time because they aren't removed or medicated by their owner, and they don't die or stop eating/defecating. *H. gallinarum* eggs can remain infective in soil for four years thus there is a high risk of transmitting blackhead to turkeys if they graze areas with chicken feces in this time frame. Thermophilic composting is known to sanitize soil from ascarid (another nematode) eggs.

The most common symptom of blackhead disease is yellow watery bird droppings. To reduce the spreading of Blackhead disease, the sick birds must be removed and their litter changed.

Intestinal Protozoa Important to Poultry

Parasites of two major groups are responsible for economic damage to poultry. These are the coccidia and related organisms, and the flagellates, including *Histomonas*, and *Trichomonas*. Complete reviews of these parasites and their control are found in Long (1982), McDougald and Reid (1978) and McDougald (1997).

Coccidia and Related Organisms

Most commonly recognised coccidia infecting chickens and other poultry are of the genus *Eimeria*. Other genera are represented, including *Toxoplasma* and *Sarcocystis*, but these are two-host parasites and rarely cause problems in commercial poultry. *Isospora* are common in wild birds. Another organism, *Cryptosporidium*, is common and widespread in chickens and turkeys, but its clinical or economic significance is unknown.

The Biology and Epidemiology of Coccidiosis

The *Eimeria* infecting chickens and turkeys do not infect other animals, nor do those of other animals infect poultry. There is a direct life cycle, not involving intermediate hosts. Spread from bird to bird and from flock to flock depends on the survival of oocysts of the parasite in the bedding or soil, where it may be eaten by another susceptible chicken.

The rigid life cycle of coccidia is a valuable tool in identifying the species of coccidia as well as the importance of an infection. Other biological characters are also useful in diagnosis and identification (McDougald, 1997). The location and appearance of lesions is very specific. The size of oocysts and the appearance of other developmental stages in microscopic smears are also helpful in determining species present.

All of the coccidia are pathogenic, although some to a lesser degree. Mortality is common with *Eimeria tenella* and Eimeria necatrix in chickens and Eimeria adenoeides, Eimeria gallopavonis, and Eimeria meleagrimitis in the turkey, but others cause reduced weight gain and wasted feed, dehydration, secondary infections, malabsorption of specific nutrients, and may potentiate other diseases. The most commonly recognised species in broiler chickens are *Eimeria acervulina*, *E. tenella*, and Eimeria maxima.

The Life Cycle of Coccidia and its Importance

Unlike bacteria and some other protozoa, the coccidia have a very strict life cycle. Oocysts ingested by the bird are crushed in the gizzard, releasing sporocysts. The action of trypsin and bile in the duodenum activates and releases sporozoites, which invade the mucosa to become trophozoites. During a preclinical phase of development, the parasites undergo a rapid multiple fission called schizogony, wherein hundreds of daughter cells are produced. These new cells, called merozoites, enter more mucosal cells and grow into second and sometimes third generation schizonts. Clinical signs are associated with tissue destruction as these forms mature. The merozoites produced by second and third generation schizonts develop into sexual forms called gametocytes, giving rise to microgametes and macrogametes.

The motile microgametes seek out and unite with the larger macrogametes in a sexual fusion, and the resulting zygote matures into a new oocyst. In this way, thousands or millions (depending on the species) of new oocysts are produced for each infecting unit.

The signs of coccidiosis can be correlated with specific stages in development. Knowledge of the life cycle can be helpful in diagnosis. The severity of lesions depends largely on the size of the exposure or number of oocysts ingested by the host. The self-regulating nature of the life cycle is used as the basis for live vaccines using nonattenuated strains, by dosage regulation.

Monitoring of Litter Oocysts

Litter oocyst monitoring can give important information if collected on a routine basis over a long period. The age of the flock when litter is sampled is extremely important, as the most oocysts will be present when the birds are 4 to 5 wk of age. Better samples can be obtained if fresh faecal droppings are used rather than whole litter.

Chemotherapy and Control

Since the 1950s, anticoccidial drugs have been used to control coccidiosis in broilers. Numerous products were introduced, many of which are available and used today. Outbreaks of coccidiosis are caused by various conditions, including 1) failure of the anticoccidial, either through drug resistance of the coccidia or inadequate spectrum of activity of the drug, 2) mismanagement or accidental application of the drug, such as low levels, mistakes in feed delivery, poor mixing, or rarely, poor product quality such as lumpy premix, 3) concurrent disease that might destroy the birds' immune system or interfere with coccidiostat intake by reduction in feed or water consumption, and 4) the mistaken diagnosis of coccidiosis when other diseases cause the same type of lesions.

Since 1971, the preferred drugs for coccidiosis prevention have been ionophorous antibiotics. There are now six products in this category, with the recent registration of semduramicin2 in the U.S.

Ionophores kill coccidia by interfering with the balance of important ions such as sodium and potassium. The host cells are able to manage these ions in the presence of ionophores, but the parasites cannot. Research has demonstrated that coccidia are destroyed by contact with the drug in the intestinal tract, and also when the drugs are absorbed into parasitised cells. Studies with fluorescein and rubidium have shown that the membranes of drug resistant coccidia are altered, and exhibit different physiological characteristics, particularly regarding esterase activity. The ionophores are unique in this type of activity, accounting for their long history of usefulness. Anticoccidials are used in various ways. Some producers use programs where an anticoccidial is used in the starter and grower feeds, and then the finisher is unmedicated. In other instances, one anticoccidial is used in the starter and another in the grower feed. This method is called a *Shuttle* or *Dual* program. Some producers actually use more than two products in this type of program, but this is not a widespread practice. If coccidiosis exposure is not high, such as in certain seasons of the year, producers may choose to reduce the length of time an anticoccidial is used. In some instances, the anticoccidial is withdrawn for two weeks. The decision to use such practices must be based on individual experience, along with the expected level of exposure for a particular locality and season.

Most producers in the U.S. use roxarsone in combination with the anticoccidial during the starting and growing periods. Roxarsone has important anticoccidial activity, particularly against *E. tenella*, and works very well in combination with ionophores. Where coccidiosis exposure is high, producers are finding that this product offers important help.

Flagellates: Histomonas and Related Organisms

Flagellates are common in the intestinal tracts of birds, but few are responsible for serious disease and economic loss. These parasites differ greatly from the Coccidia in their biology, phylogeny, and ultimately, methods of treatment or control. Commonly reported from poultry are 1) Histomonas meleagridis, 2) Trichomonas spp. and 3) *Giardia* spp.

Blackhead Disease

The parasite causing Blackhead Disease has a surprisingly complicated life cycle involving intermediate hosts and carriers. Turkeys are especially susceptible to infection. If left untreated, more than 90% of infected birds may die. Chickens are less susceptible, but flocks of breeder pullets may suffer high morbidity and mortality of 10 to 20%, with increased culling and poor uniformity of layers. Recent increases in outbreaks of blackhead in broiler breeder pullets seem to be related to destruction of the T cell system by other (sometimes unknown) infections. The blackhead organism, *Histomonas meleagridis*, is very sensitive to environmental conditions outside the host, and are carried from host to host by eggs of the cecal worm *Heterakis gallinarum*. Encased in heterakis eggs, the histomonads may remain viable for years in suitable conditions in soil, or in earthworms, which may consume the eggs along with soil. Lateral transmission is possible during heavy infections, although the organisms will not remain viable for long outside the host.

Diagnosis of Blackhead Disease depends on the observation of lesions in the ceca or liver (McDougald, 1997). Cecal infections are characterised by whitish to yellow caseous cores. The mucosa may be thickened and inflamed. Mesenteries and blood vessels around the ceca and intestines are inflamed. Lesions may also occur in the liver, and vary widely in appearance, from wellcircumscribed, sunken, necrotic foci, to subsurface light mottling. Confirmatory microscopic observation of the protozoa in the ceca or liver can be made with high power (220 to 440´) microscopy. *Histomonas meleagridis* can readily be cultured *in vitro* using a simple medium (McDougald and Galloway, 1973).

Control and Treatment of Blackhead Disease. Until recently, Blackhead Disease could be treated with nitroimidazoles, such as dimetridazole or ipronidazole. Currently, no products are sold in the U.S. for treatment of Blackhead. Metronidazole, which is used in human medicine, has some effectiveness against Blackhead and other flagellate infections, but would be expensive for treatment of flocks of commercial poultry.

To some extent, prevention of Blackhead is improved by better control of cecal worms. Use hygromicin b in feed throughout the early growth of pullets. Levamisole is reportedly used for periodic treatment to eliminate worm infections.

Trichomonas and other Flagellates

Several species of *Trichomonas* infect commercial and noncommercial birds. Most infections are symptomless, although some highly virulent strains are known. All pigeons are infected with *Trichomonas gallinae*. Other Protozoa found in the intestinal tract of birds include Tetratrichomonas gallinarum, Chilomastix gallinarum, Cochlosoma *anatis*, and *Hexamita meleagridis*. Little is known about these parasites. Occasional outbreaks of *Hexamita* are reported, but there has been no research on these organisms in many years.

Histomoniasis is caused by a protozoan parasite named Histomonas meleagridis. Often called blackhead disease, histomoniasis primarily affects gallinaceous birds (chickens, grouse, partridge, peafowl, pheasants, quail, turkeys). The old name "blackhead disease" is a misnomer because the heads of birds infected with histomoniasis do not turn black. Despite the limited number of confirmed reports, histomoniasis is an important disease of wild turkeys.

Signs of Infection

Clinical signs in turkeys may include sulfur-coloured droppings, lethargy, drooping wings, eyes closed, head held close to the body, weakness, or emaciation. Lesions are characterised by thickening and ulceration of the lining of the ceca and by focal necrosis in the liver. The combination of swollen, inflamed ceca with yellow, cheesy cecal cores and discrete spots of necrosis in the liver is considered indicative for histomoniasis. Variations in the severity and appearance of lesions are not uncommon, however, and cecal lesions without liver involvement occur occasionally.

NWTF Wildlife Bulletin No.25 Nationalwild Turkey Federation Glenn C. Smith

A healthy wild turkey gobbler in full strut looking for a mate. Histomoniasis appears frequently in the scientific, semi-technical, and popular literature in discussions of diseases of wild turkeys; however, scientifically confirmed accounts of histomoniasis in wild turkeys are relatively few. For example, it accounted for 12% of 266 sick or dead wild turkeys from 10 southeastern states that were submitted for diagnosis to the Southeastern Cooperative Wildlife Disease Study on the University of Georgia/Athens campus from 1972-1994.

Different species of galliform birds vary greatly in their susceptibility to clinical disease due to histomoniasis.

The course of infection in different host species spans the entire spectrum from a total tolerance without lesions to severe disease with a very high death rate.

Unfortunately, turkeys, either wild or domestic, almost always develop severe disease following infection. Chukar partridge, peafowl and ruffed grouse also are prone to severe disease. At the opposite end of the spectrum are species such as ring-necked pheasants.

Gary Doster

The cheesy core in the ceca of a turkey infected with histomoniasis.

Gary Doster

The liver of a turkey infected with histomoniasis. Note the discoloured, depressed lesions. junglefowl which rarely become sick; these species serve as carriers of the parasite for more susceptible species such as wild turkeys. Bobwhites, guinea fowl and Hungarian partridge occupy intermediate positions in which clinical disease is common, but with fewer instances of sickness or death. Aside from the fact that diseased avian hosts may die and be lost as a source of infection, survival of the heterakid roundworm vector in diseased ceca is extremely poor and often the worms die before the birds do. Thus, individual birds or species in which severe cecal lesions develop usually are not important sources for transmission. In contrast, hosts in which cecal lesions are absent or minimal continue to support heterakids which in turn produce large numbers of histomonad- bearing eggs.

Wild Turkeys, Pheasants and Chickens Don't Mix

These epidemiologic factors are important considerations in the prevention and control of histomoniasis under field conditions. They serve as the basis of the old axiom of poultry producers "do not raise chickens and turkeys together."

They also form the basis for the recommendations in place for many decades not to introduce "carrier" species such as pheasants or junglefowl into habitats occupied by wild turkeys and not to use chicken litter as fertilizer on fields or pastures frequented by wild turkeys.

Concepts regarding the disease risk posed to wild birds by the use of chicken litter as fertilizer were derived long before modern improvements in husbandry and disease control within the commercial poultry industry.

Dave Menke/Usfws

"Carrier" species, like this ring-necked pheasant should not be introduced into habitats already occupied by wild turkey populations.

The histomanads invade the lining of the ceca, producing thickening, ulceration, and hemorrhage, which are accompanied by extensive inflammation and the development of cheese cecal cores.

Histomonads from the cecal lesions commonly gain entry to small veins and are carried by the blood to the liver. In the liver the histomonads continue reproducing and cause focal areas of necrosis and an intense inflammatory response. A diagnosis of histomoniasis can best be made upon examination of a fresh, refrigerated carcass. However, if it is not possible to deliver the carcass to a diagnostic laboratory within 2 or 3 days after death, a frozen carcass can be used. The way that Histomoniasis meleagridis is transmitted from bird to bird is unusual in that it is dependent upon a parasitic roundworm, Heterakis gallinarum, which also infects the ceca of many species of galliform birds. The histomonads, in addition to infecting the ceca of the bird, also infect the female heterakid worms and become incorporated within the worm's eggs.

The delicate histomonads, which do not survive direct exposure to the environment, are transmitted within the protective covering of worm eggs in the droppings of infected birds. When the histomonad-bearing worm eggs are ingested by a suitable host and hatch, the histomonads are released in the ceca where they reproduce by repeated division. Birds also may acquire both heterakid worms and histomonads by consuming earthworms which can serve as transport hosts of heterakid larvae by ingesting heterakid larvae and in this capacity as transport hosts are an important means of transmission, especially under field conditions.

Botulism

Botulism (Latin, *botulus*, "sausage") also known as botulinus intoxication is a rare but serious paralytic illness caused by botulinum toxin which is metabolic waste produced under anaerobic conditions by the bacterium *Clostridium botulinum*, and affecting a wide range of mammals, birds and fish.

The toxin enters the human body in one of three ways: by colonisation of the digestive tract by the bacterium in children (infant botulism) or adults (adult intestinal toxemia), by ingestion of toxin from foods (foodborne botulism) or by contamination of a wound by the bacterium (wound botulism). Person to person transmission of botulism does not occur.

All forms lead to paralysis that typically starts with the muscles of the face and then spreads towards the limbs. In severe forms, it leads to paralysis of the breathing muscles and causes respiratory failure. In view of this life-threatening complication, all suspected cases of botulism are treated as medical emergencies, and public health officials are usually involved to prevent further cases from the same source.

Botulism can be prevented by killing the spores by pressure cooking or autoclaving at 121 °C (250 °F) for 3 minutes or providing conditions that prevent the spores from growing. The toxin itself is destroyed by normal cooking processes - that is, boiling for a few minutes. Additional precautions for infants include not feeding them honey.

Signs and Symptoms

Clinical Features

The muscle weakness of botulism characteristically starts in the muscles supplied by the cranial nerves. A group of twelve nerves controls eye movements, the facial muscles and the muscles controlling chewing and swallowing. Double vision, drooping of both eyelids, loss of facial expression and swallowing problems may therefore occur, as well as difficulty with talking. The weakness then spreads to the arms (starting in the shoulders and proceeding to the forearms) and legs (again from the thighs down to the feet). Severe botulism leads to reduced movement of the muscles of respiration, and hence problems with gas exchange. This may be experienced as dyspnea (difficulty breathing), but when severe can lead to respiratory failure, due to the buildup of unexhaled carbon dioxide and its resultant depressant effect on the brain. This may lead to coma and eventually death if untreated. In addition to affecting the voluntary muscles, it can also cause disruptions in the autonomic nervous system. This is experienced as a dry mouth and throat (due to decreased production of saliva), postural hypotension (decreased blood pressure on standing, with resultant lightheadedness and risk of blackouts), and eventually constipation (due to decreased peristalsis). Some of the toxins (B and E) also precipitate nausea and vomiting.

Clinicians frequently think of the symptoms of botulism in terms of a classic triad: bulbar palsy and descending paralysis, lack of fever, and clear senses and mental status ("clear sensorium").

Mode of Acquisition

Four main modes of entry for the toxin are known. The most common form in Western countries is *infant botulism*. This occurs in small children who are colonised with the bacterium during the early stages of their lives. The bacterium then releases the toxin into the intestine, which is absorbed into the bloodstream. The consumption of honey during the first year of life has been identified as a risk factor for infant botulism; it is a factor in a fifth of all cases. The adult form of infant botulism is termed *adult intestinal toxemia*, and is exceedingly rare.

Foodborne botulism results from contaminated foodstuffs in which *C. botulinum* spores have been allowed to germinate in anaerobic conditions. This typically occurs in home-canned food substances and fermented uncooked dishes. Given that multiple people often consume food from the same source, it is common for more than a single person to be affected simultaneously. Symptoms usually appear 12–36 hours after eating, but can also appear within 6 hours to 10 days.

Wound botulism results from the contamination of a wound with the bacteria, which then secrete the toxin into the bloodstream. This has become more common in intravenous drug users since the 1990s, especially people using black tar heroin and those injecting heroin into the skin rather than the veins.

Isolated cases of botulism have been described after inhalation by laboratory workers and after cosmetic use of inappropriate strengths of Botox.

Infant Botulism

Infant botulism was first recognised in 1976, and is the most common form of botulism in the United States. There are 80 - 100 diagnosed cases of infant botulism in the United States each year. Infants are susceptible to infant botulism in the first year of life, with more than 90% of cases occurring in infants younger than six months. Infant botulism results from the ingestion of the *C. botulinum* spores, and subsequent colonisation of the small intestine. The infant gut may be colonised when the composition of the intestinal microflora (normal flora) is insufficient to competitively inhibit the growth of *C. botulinum*. Medical science does not yet completely understand all factors that make an infant susceptible to *C. botulinum* colonisation. The growth of the spores releases botulinum toxin, which is then absorbed into the bloodstream and taken throughout the body, causing paralysis by blocking the release of acetylcholine at the neuromuscular junction. Typical symptoms of infant botulism include constipation, lethargy, weakness, difficulty feeding and an altered cry, often progressing to a complete descending flaccid paralysis. Although constipation is usually the first symptom of infant botulism, it is commonly overlooked.

Honey is the only known dietary reservoir of *C. botulinum* spores linked to infant botulism. For this reason honey should not be fed to infants less than one year of age. Due to the success of this public health message, fewer than 5% of recent infant botulism cases have been exposed to honey. The remaining 95% of infant botulism cases are thought to have acquired the spores from the natural environment. *Clostridium botulinum* is a ubiquitous soil-dwelling bacterium. Many infant botulism patients have been demonstrated to live near a construction site or an area of soil disturbance.

Infant botulism has been reported in 49 of 50 US states, and cases have been recognised in 26 countries on five continents.

Complications

Infant botulism has no long-term side effects, but can be complicated by nosocomial adverse events. The case fatality rate is less than 1% for hospitalised infants with botulism.

Botulism can result in death due to respiratory failure. However, in the past 50 years, the proportion of patients with botulism who die has fallen from about 50% to 8% due to improved supportive care. A patient with severe botulism may require a breathing machine as well as intensive medical and nursing care for several months. Patients who survive an episode of botulism poisoning may have fatigue and shortness of breath for years and long-term therapy may be needed to aid their recovery.

Mechanism

C. botulinum is an anaerobic, Gram positive, spore-forming rod. Botulin toxin is one of the most powerful known toxins: about one microgram is lethal to humans. It acts by blocking nerve function and leads to respiratory and musculoskeletal paralysis.

In all cases illness is caused by the toxin made by *C. botulinum,* not by the bacterium itself. The pattern of damage occurs because the toxin affects nerves that are firing more often. Specifically, the toxin acts by blocking the production or release of acetylcholine at synapses and neuromuscular junctions. Death occurs due to respiratory failure.

Diagnosis

For infant botulism, diagnosis should be made on clinical grounds. Confirmation of the diagnosis is made by testing of a stool or enema specimen with the mouse bioassay.

Physicians may consider diagnosing botulism if the patient's history and physical examination suggest botulism. However, these clues are often not enough to allow a diagnosis. Other diseases such as Guillain-Barré syndrome, stroke, and myasthenia gravis can appear similar to botulism, and special tests may be needed to exclude these other conditions. These tests may include a brain scan, cerebrospinal fluid examination, nerve conduction test (electromyography, or EMG), and an edrophonium chloride (Tensilon) test for myasthenia gravis. A definite diagnosis can be made if botulinum toxin is identified in the food, stomach or intestinal contents, vomit or feces. The toxin is occasionally found in the blood in peracute cases. Botulinum toxin can be detected by a variety of techniques, including enzyme-linked immunosorbent assays (ELISAs), electrochemiluminescent (ECL) tests and mouse inoculation or feeding trials. The toxins can be typed with neutralisation tests in mice. In toxicoinfectious botulism, the organism can be cultured from tissues. On egg yolk medium, toxin-producing colonies usually display surface iridescence that extends beyond the colony.

In cattle, the symptoms may include drooling, restlessness, uncoordination, urine retention, dysphagia, and sternal recumbency. Laterally recumbent animals are usually very close to death. In sheep, the symptoms may include drooling, a serous nasal discharge, stiffness, and incoordination. Abdominal respiration may be observed and the tail may switch on the side. As the disease progresses, the limbs may become paralysed and death may occur. Phosphorus-deficient cattle, especially in southern Africa, are inclined to ingest bones and carrion containing clostridial toxins and consequently suffer *lame sickness* or *lamsiekte*.

The clinical signs in horses are similar to cattle. The muscle paralysis is progressive; it usually begins at the hindquarters and gradually moves to the front limbs, neck, and head. Death generally occurs 24 to 72 hours after initial symptoms and results from respiratory paralysis. Some foals are found dead without other clinical signs.

Pigs are relatively resistant to botulism. Reported symptoms include anorexia, refusal to drink, vomiting, pupillary dilation, and muscle paralysis.

In poultry and wild birds, flaccid paralysis is usually seen in the legs, wings, neck and eyelids. Broiler chickens with the toxicoinfectious form may also have diarrhea with excess urates.

Prevention

Although the botulinum toxin is destroyed by thorough cooking over the course of a few minutes, the spore itself is not killed by the temperatures reached with normal sea-level-pressure boiling, leaving it free to grow and again produce the toxin when conditions are right.

A recommended prevention measure for infant botulism is to avoid feeding honey to infants less than 12 months of age. In older children and adults the normal intestinal bacteria suppress development of *C. botulinum.*

While commercially canned goods are required to undergo a "botulinum cook" in a pressure cooker at 121 °C (250 °F) for 3 minutes, and so rarely cause botulism, there have been notable exceptions such as the 1978 Alaskan salmon outbreak and the 2007 Castleberry's Food Company outbreak.

Foodborne botulism is the rarest form though, accounting for only around 15% of cases (US) and has more frequently been from home-canned foods with low acid content, such as carrot juice, asparagus, green beans, beets, and corn. However, outbreaks of botulism have resulted from more unusual sources. In July, 2002, fourteen Alaskans ate *muktuk* (whale meat) from a beached whale, and eight of them developed symptoms of botulism, two of them requiring mechanical ventilation.

Other, but much rarer sources of infection (about every decade in the US) include garlic or herbs stored covered in oil without acidification, chilli peppers, improperly handled baked potatoes wrapped in aluminium foil, tomatoes, and home-canned or fermented fish. Persons who do home canning should follow strict hygienic procedures to reduce contamination of foods. Oils infused with fresh garlic or herbs should be acidified and refrigerated. Potatoes which have been baked while wrapped in aluminum foil should be kept hot until served or refrigerated. Because the botulism toxin is destroyed by high temperatures, home-canned foods are best boiled for 10 minutes before eating. Metal cans containing food in which bacteria, possibly botulinum, are growing may bulge outwards due to gas production from bacterial growth; such cans should be discarded. Any container of food which has been heat-treated and then assumed to be airtight which shows signs of not being so, e.g., metal cans with pinprick holes from rust or mechanical damage, should also be discarded. Contamination of a canned food solely with *C. botulinum* may not cause any visual defects (e.g. bulging). Only sufficient thermal processing during production should be used as a food safety control.

Wound botulism can be prevented by promptly seeking medical care for infected wounds, and by avoiding punctures by unsterile things such as needles used for street drug injections. It is currently being researched at USAMRIID under BSL-434.

Treatment

Most infant botulism patients require supportive care in a hospital setting. The only drug currently available to treat infant botulism is Botulism Immune Globulin Intravenous-Human (BIG-IV or BabyBIG). BabyBIG was developed by the Infant Botulism Treatment and Prevention Program at the California Department of Public Health.

The respiratory failure and paralysis that occur with severe botulism may require a patient to be on a ventilator for weeks, plus intensive medical and nursing care. After several weeks, the paralysis slowly improves. If diagnosed early, foodborne and wound botulism can be treated by inducing passive immunity with a horse-derived antitoxin, which blocks the action of toxin circulating in the blood. This can prevent patients from worsening, but recovery still takes many weeks. Physicians may try to remove contaminated food still in the gut by inducing vomiting or by using enemas. Wounds should be treated, usually surgically, to remove the source of the toxin-producing bacteria. Good supportive care in a hospital is the mainstay of therapy for all forms of botulism.

Furthermore each case of food-borne botulism is a potential public health emergency in that it is necessary to identify the source of the outbreak and ensure that all persons who have been exposed to the toxin have been identified, and that no contaminated food remains. There are two primary Botulinum Antitoxins available for treatment of wound and foodborne botulism. Trivalent (A,B,E) Botulinum Antitoxin is derived from equine sources utilising whole antibodies (Fab & Fc portions).

This antitoxin is available from the local health department via the CDC. The second antitoxin is heptavalent (A,B,C,D,E,F,G) Botulinum Antitoxin which is derived from "despeciated" equine IgG antibodies which have had the Fc portion cleaved off leaving the F(ab')2 portions. This is a less immunogenic antitoxin that is effective against all known strains of botulism where not contraindicated. This is available from the US Army. On 1 June 2006 the US Department of Health and Human Services awarded a $363 million contract with Cangene Corporation for 200,000 doses of Heptavalent Botulinum Antitoxin over five years for delivery into the Strategic National Stockpile beginning in 2007.

Prognosis

Infant botulism has no long-term side effects, but can be complicated by nosocomial adverse events. The case fatality rate is less than 1% for hospitalised infants with botulism.

Between 1910 and 1919 the death rate from botulism was 70% in the United States, dropping to 9% in the 1980s and 2% in the early 1990s, mainly because of the development of artificial respirators. Up to 60% of botulism cases are fatal if left untreated.

The World Health Organisation (WHO) reports that the current mortality rate is 5% (type B) to 10% (type A). Other sources report that, in the U.S., the overall mortality rate is about 7.5%, but the mortality rate among adults over 60 is 30%. The mortality rate for wound botulism is about 10%. The infant botulism mortality rate is about 1.3%.

Death from botulism is common in waterfowl; an estimated 10,000 to 100,000 birds die of botulism annually. In some large outbreaks, a million or more birds may die. Ducks appear to be affected most often. Botulism also affects commercially raised poultry. In chickens, the mortality rate varies from a few birds to 40% of the flock. Some affected birds may recover without treatment.

Botulism seems to be relatively uncommon in domestic mammals; however, in some parts of the world, epidemics with up to 65% mortality are seen in cattle. The prognosis is poor in large animals that are recumbent. Most dogs with botulism recover within 2 weeks.

Epidemiology

Between 1990 and 2000, the Centres for Disease Control reported 263 individual 'cases' from 160 foodborne botulism 'events' in the United States with a case-fatality rate of 4%. Thirty-nine percent (103 cases and 58 events) occurred in Alaska, all of which were attributable to traditional Alaska aboriginal foods. In the lower 49 states, home-canned food was implicated in 70 (91%) events with canned asparagus being the most numerous cause. Two restaurant-associated outbreaks affected 25 persons. The median number of cases per year was 23 (range 17–43), the median number of events per year was 14 (range 9–24). The highest incidence rates occurred in Alaska, Idaho, Washington, and Oregon. All other states had an incidence rate of 1 case per ten million people or less.

The number of cases of food borne and infant botulism has changed little in recent years, but wound botulism has increased because of the use of black tar heroin, especially in California.

Outbreaks

Castleberry's Food Company Outbreak

Beginning in late June 2007, 8 people contracted botulism poisoning by eating canned food products produced by Castleberry's Food Company in its Augusta, Georgia plant. It was later identified that the Castleberry's plant had serious production issues on a specific line of retorts that had under-processed the cans of food. These issues included broken cooking alarms, leaking water valves and inaccurate temperature devices, all the result of poor management of the company.

All of the victims were hospitalised and placed on mechanical ventilation. The Castleberry's Food Company outbreak was the first instance of botulism in commercial canned foods in the United States in over 30 years.

Bon Vivant incident

On July 2, 1971, the U.S. Food and Drug Administration (FDA) released a public warning after learning that a New York man had died and his wife had become seriously ill due to botulism after eating a can of Bon Vivant vichyssoise soup.

In other Species

Botulism can occur in many vertebrates and invertebrates are reports are not just limited to humans, rats, mouse, chicken, frogs, toads, goldfish, aplysia, squid, crayfish, drosophila, leech etc.

Campylobacteriosis

Campylobacteriosis is an infection by the *Campylobacter* bacterium, most commonly *C. jejuni*. It is among the most common bacterial infections of humans, often a foodborne illness. It produces an inflammatory, sometimes bloody, diarrhea or dysentery syndrome, mostly including cramps, fever and pain.

Cause

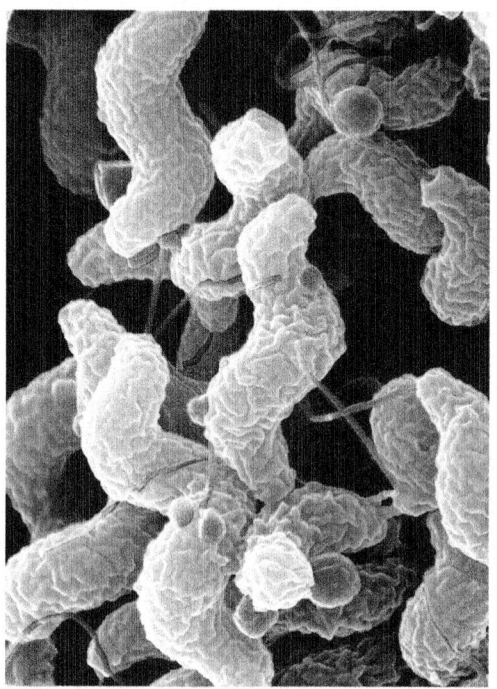

Figure : Campylobacter bacteria are the number-one cause of food-related gastrointestinal illness in the United States. This scanning electron microscope image shows the characteristic spiral, or corkscrew, shape of C. jejuni cells and related structures.

Campylobacteriosis is caused by *Campylobacter* organisms. These are curved or spiral, motile, non–spore-forming, Gram-negative rods. This is most commonly caused by *C. jejuni*, a spiral and comma shaped bacterium normally found in cattle, swine, and birds, where it is nonpathogenic, but the illness can also be caused by *C. coli* (also found in cattle, swine, and birds), *C. upsaliensis* (found in cats and dogs) and *C. lari* (present in seabirds in particular). One effect of campylobacteriosis is tissue injury in the gut. The sites of tissue injury include the jejunum, the ileum, and the colon. *C jejuni* appears to achieve this by invading and destroying epithelial cells.

C. jejuni can also cause a latent autoimmune effect on the nerves of the legs, which is usually seen several weeks after a surgical procedure of the adomen. The effect is known as an acute idiopathic demyelinating polyneuropathy (AIDP), i.e. Guillain-Barre syndrome, in which one sees symptoms of ascending paralysis, dysaesthesias usually below the waist, and, in the later stages, respiratory failure.

Some strains of *C jejuni* produce a cholera-like enterotoxin, which is important in the watery diarrhea observed in infections. The organism produces diffuse, bloody, edematous, and exudative enteritis. In a small number of cases, the infection may be associated with hemolytic uremic syndrome and thrombotic thrombocytopenic purpura through a poorly understood mechanism.

Transmission

The common routes of transmission for the disease-causing bacteria are faecal-oral, person-to-person sexual contact, ingestion of contaminated food (generally unpasteurised (raw) milk and undercooked or poorly handled poultry), and waterborne (i.e., through contaminated drinking water). Contact with contaminated poultry, livestock, or household pets, especially puppies, can also cause disease. Animals farmed for meat are the main source of campylobacteriosis. A study published in PLoS Genetics (September 26, 2008) by researchers from Lancashire, England, and Chicago, IL, found that 97 percent of campylobacteriosis cases sampled in Lancashire were caused by bacteria typically found in chicken and livestock. In 57 percent of cases, the bacteria could be traced to chicken, and in 35 percent to cattle. Wild animal and environmental sources were accountable for just three percent of disease.

The infectious dose is 1000-10,000 bacteria (although ten to five hundred bacteria can be enough to infect humans). *Campylobacter* species are sensitive to hydrochloric acid in the stomach, and acid reduction treatment can reduce the amount of inoculum needed to cause disease.

Exposure to bacteria is often more common during travelling, and therefore campylobacteriosis is a common form of travellers' diarrhea.

Epidemiology

Infection with a *Campylobacter* species is one of the most common causes of human bacterial gastroenteritis. For instance, an estimated 2 million cases of *Campylobacter* enteritis occur annually in the U.S., accounting for 5-7% of cases of gastroenteritis. Furthermore, in the United Kingdom during 2000, *Campylobacter jejuni* was involved in 77.3% in all cases of foodborne illness. About 15 of every 100,000 people are diagnosed with campylobacteriosis every year, and with many cases going unreported, up to 0.5% of the general population may unknowingly harbour *Campylobacter* in their gut.

A large animal reservoir is present as well, with up to 100% of poultry, including chickens, turkeys, and waterfowl, having asymptomatic infections in their intestinal tracts. Infected chicken feces may contain up to 10^9 bacteria per 25 grams, and due to the installations, the bacteria are rapidly spread to other chickens. This vastly exceeds the infectious dose of 1000-10,000 bacteria for humans.

Symptoms

The prodrome is fever, headache, and myalgias, lasting as long as 24 hours. The actual latent period is 2–5 days (sometimes 1–6 days). In other words, it typically takes 1–2 days until actual symptoms develop. These are diarrhea (as many as 10 watery, frequently bloody, bowel movements per day) or dysentery, cramps, abdominal pain, and fever as high as 40°C (104°F). In most people, the illness lasts for 2–10 days. This is classified as invasive/inflammatory diarrhea, also known as bloody diarrhea or dysentry.

Symptoms may also depend on route of transmission. In participants of anal intercourse, campylobacteriosis is more localised to the distal end of the colon and may be termed a proctocolitis.

There are other diseases showing similar symptoms. For instance, abdominal pain and tenderness may be very localised, mimicking acute appendicitis. Furthermore, *Helicobacter pylori* is closely related to Campylobacter and causes peptic ulcer disease.

Other Factors

In patients with HIV, infections may be more frequent, may cause prolonged bouts of dirty brown diarrhea, and may be more commonly associated with bacteremia and antibiotic resistance. The severity and persistence of infection in patients with AIDS and hypogammaglobulinemia indicates that both cell-mediated and humoral immunity are important in preventing and terminating infection.

Diagnosis

Campylobacter organisms can be detected by performing a Gram stain of a stool sample with high specificity and a sensitivity of ~60%, but are most often diagnosed by stool culture. faecal leukocytes should be present and indicate the diarrhea to be inflammatory in nature. Methods currently being developed to detect the presence of campylobacter organisms include antigen testing via an EIA or PCR.

Treatment

The infection is usually self-limiting, and in most cases, symptomatic treatment by liquid and electrolyte replacement is enough in human infections.

Antibiotics

Antibiotic treatment is controversial, and has only a marginal benefit (1.32 days) on the duration of symptoms, and should not be used routinely.

Erythromycin can be used in children, and tetracycline in adults. Some studies show, however, that erythromycin rapidly eliminates *Campylobacter* from the stool without affecting the duration of illness. Nevertheless, children with dysentery due to *C. jejuni* benefit from early treatment with erythromycin. Treatment with antibiotics, therefore, depends on the severity of symptoms. Quinolones are effective if the organism is sensitive, but high rates of quinolone use in livestock means that quinolones are now largely ineffective. Antimotility agents, such as loperamide, can lead to prolonged illness or intestinal perforation in any invasive diarrhea, and should be avoided. Trimethoprim-sulfamethoxazole and ampicillin are ineffective against *Campylobacter*.

In Animals

In the past, poultry infections were often treated by mass administration of enrofloxacin and sarafloxacin for single instances of infection. The FDA banned this practice, as it promoted the development of fluoroquinolone-resistant populations. A major broad-spectrum fluoroquinolone used in humans is ciprofloxacin.

Currently growing resistance of the *Campylobacter* to fluoroquinolones and macrolides is of a major concern.

Prognosis

Campylobacteriosis is usually self-limited without any mortality. However, there are several possible complications.

Complications

Some (1-2 in 100,000 cases) individuals develop Guillain-Barré syndrome, in which the nerves that join the spinal cord and brain to the rest of the body are damaged, sometimes permanently. This occurs only with infection of *C. jejuni* and *C. upsaliensis*.

Other complications include toxic megacolon, dehydration and sepsis. Such complications generally form in little children (< 1 year of age) and immunocompromised people. A chronic course of the disease is possible; such form of the process is likely to develop without a distinct acute phase. Chronic campylobacteriosis features long period of sub-febrile temperature and asthenia; eye damage, arthritis, endocarditis may develop if infection is untreated.

Occasional deaths occur in young, previously healthy individuals because of blood volume depletion, and in persons who are elderly or immunocompromised.

A mysterious paralysis can attack people who just had mild symptoms of campylobacteriosis years earlier.

Prevention

Pasteurisation of milk and chlorination of drinking water destroy the organism.

Treatment with antibiotics can reduce faecal excretion.

Infected health care workers should not provide direct patient care. Separate cutting boards should be used for foods of animal origin and other foods. After preparing raw food of animal origin, all cutting boards and countertops should be carefully cleaned with soap and hot water.

Contact with pet saliva and feces should be avoided.

Following are recommendations of the World Health Organisation.

Recommendations for the public and travellers - Your food should be properly cooked and hot when served.

Consume only pasteurised or boiled milk and milk products, never raw milk products.

Make sure that ice is from safe water. If you are not sure of the safety of drinking water, boil it, or disinfect it with chemical disinfectant.

Wash hands thoroughly and frequently with soap, especially after using the toilet and after contact with pets and farm animals.

Wash fruits and vegetables thoroughly, especially if they are to be eaten raw. Peel fruits and vegetables whenever possible.

Recommendations for Food Handlers

Food handlers, professionals and at home, should observe hygenic rules during food preparation. Professional food handlers should immediately report to their employer any fever, diarrhoea, vomiting or visible infected skin lesions.

Campylobacter

Classification and external resources

ICD-10	A04.5
ICD-9	008.43
DiseasesDB	1914
MedlinePlus	000224
eMedicine	ped/2697 med/263
MeSH	D002169

Campylobacter (meaning 'twisted bacteria') is a genus of bacteria that are Gram-negative, spiral, and microaerophilic. Motile, with either unipolar or bipolar flagella, the organisms have a characteristic spiral/corkscrew appearance and are oxidase-positive. *Campylobacter jejuni* is now recognised as one of the main causes of bacterial foodborne disease in many developed countries. At least a dozen species of *Campylobacter* have been implicated in human disease, with *C. jejuni* and *C. coli* the most common. *C. fetus* is a cause of spontaneous abortions in cattle and sheep, as well as an opportunistic pathogen in humans. Recommendations for food handlers

Genome

The genomes of several *Campylobacter* species have been sequenced, providing insights into their mechanisms of pathogenesis.

The first *Campylobacter* genome to be sequenced was *C. jejuni*, in 2000.

Campylobacter species contain two flagellin genes in tandem for motility, *flaA* and *flaB*. These genes undergo intergenic recombination, further contributing to their virulence. Nonmotile mutants do not colonise.

Pathogenesis

Campylobacteriosis is an infection by *Campylobacter*. The common routes of transmission are faecal-oral, ingestion of contaminated food or water, and the eating of raw meat. It produces an inflammatory, sometimes bloody, diarrhea, periodontitis or dysentery syndrome, mostly including cramps, fever and pain. The infection is usually self-limiting and in most cases, symptomatic treatment by reposition of liquid and electrolyte replacement is enough in human infections. The use of antibiotics, on the other hand, is controversial. Symptoms typically last for five to seven days.

Cause

The sites of tissue injury include the jejunum, the ileum, and the colon. Most strains of *C jejuni* produce a toxin (cytolethal distending toxin) that hinders the cells from dividing and activating the immune system. This helps the bacteria to evade the immune system and survive for a limited time in the cells. It was thought previously that a cholera-like enterotoxin was also made, but this appears not to be the case. The organism produces diffuse, bloody, edematous, and exudative enteritis. In a small number of cases, the infection may be associated with hemolytic uremic syndrome and thrombotic thrombocytopenic purpura through a poorly understood mechanism. Gastrointestinal perforation is a rare complication of ileal infection

Treatment

Diagnosis of the illness is made by testing a specimen of faeces (bowel motion).

Generally, there is little treatment apart from rest and keeping up fluid intake.

Sometimes antibiotics will be prescribed.

Dehydrated children may require intravenous (by vein) fluid treatment in a hospital.

The illness is contagious, and children must be kept at home until they have been clear of symptoms for at least two days. Good hygiene is important to avoid contracting the illness or spreading it to others. Intestinal perforation is very rare; increased abdominal pain and collapse require immediate medical attention.

History

The symptoms of *Campylobacter* infections were described in 1886 in infants by Theodour Escherich. These infections were named cholera infantum, or summer complaint. The genus was first discovered in 1963; however, the organism was not isolated until 1972.

Periodontitis

"Pyorrhea" redirects here. For the Polish band.

Periodontal Disease

Classification and External Resources

This radiograph shows significant bone loss between the two roots of a tooth (black region). The spongy bone has receded due to infection under tooth, reducing the bony support for the tooth.

Periodontitis

Periodontitis is a set of inflammatory diseases affecting the periodontium, i.e., the tissues that surround and support the teeth. Periodontitis involves progressive loss of the alveolar bone around the teeth, and if left untreated, can lead to the loosening and subsequent loss of teeth. Periodontitis is caused by microorganisms that adhere to and grow on the tooth's surfaces, along with an overly aggressive immune response against these microorganisms. A diagnosis of periodontitis is established by inspecting the soft gum tissues around the teeth with a probe (i.e. a *clinical exam*) and by evaluating the patient's x-ray films (i.e. a *radiographic exam*), to determine the amount of bone loss around the teeth. Specialists in the treatment of periodontitis are periodontists; their field is known as "periodontology" or "periodontics". The word "periodontitis" comes from *peri* ("around"), *odont* ("tooth") and *-itis* ("inflammation").

Classification

The 1999 classification system for periodontal diseases and conditions listed seven major categories of periodontal diseases, of which the last six are termed *destructive* periodontal disease because they are essentially irreversible. The seven categories are as follows:

- Gingivitis
- Chronic periodontitis
- Aggressive periodontitis
- Periodontitis as a manifestation of systemic disease
- Necrotising ulcerative gingivitis/periodontitis
- Abscesses of the periodontium
- Combined periodontic-endodontic lesions.

Moreover, terminology expressing both the extent and severity of periodontal diseases are appended to the terms above to denote the specific diagnosis of a particular patient or group of patients.

Extent

The *extent* of disease refers to the proportion of the dentition affected by the disease in terms of percentage of sites. Sites are defined as the positions at which probing measurements are taken around each tooth and, generally, six probing sites around each tooth are recorded, as follows:

- mesiobuccal
- mid-buccal
- distobuccal
- mesiolingual
- mid-lingual
- distolingual.

If up to 30% of sites in the mouth are affected, the manifestation is classification as *localised*; for more than 30%, the term *generalised* is used.

Severity

The *severity* of disease refers to the amount of periodontal ligament fibres that have been lost, termed *clinical attachment loss*. According to the American Academy of Periodontology, the classification of severity is as follows:

- *Mild*: 1–2 mm of attachment loss
- *Moderate*: 3–4 mm of attachment loss
- *Severe*: e" 5 mm of attachment lo.

Signs and Symptoms

In the early stages, periodontitis has very few symptoms and in many individuals the disease has progressed significantly before they seek treatment. Symptoms may include the following:

Redness or bleeding of gums while brushing teeth, using dental floss or biting into hard food (e.g. apples) (though this may occur even in gingivitis, where there is no attachment loss):

- Gum swelling that recurs spiting out blood after brusing teeth
- Halitosis, or bad breath, and a persistent metallic taste in the mouth.

Gingival recession, resulting in apparent lengthening of teeth. (This may also be caused by heavy handed brushing or with a stiff tooth brush.) Deep pockets between the teeth and the gums (pockets are sites where the attachment has been gradually destroyed by collagen-destroying enzymes, known as *collagenases*) Loose teeth, in the later stages (though this may occur for other reasons as well).

Patients should realise that the gingival inflammation and bone destruction are largely painless. Hence, people may wrongly assume that painless bleeding after teeth cleaning is insignificant, although this may be a symptom of progressing periodontitis in that patient.

Effects Outside the Mouth

Periodontitis has been linked to increased inflammation in the body such as indicated by raised levels of C-reactive protein and Interleukin. It is through this linked to increased risk of stroke, myocardial infarction, and atherosclerosis. It also linked in those over 60 years of age to impairments in delayed memory and calculation abilities. Individuals with impaired fasting glucose and diabetes mellitus have higher degree of periodontal inflammation, and often have difficulties with balancing their blood glucose level owing to the constant systemic inflammatory state, caused by the periodontal inflammation. Although no causative connection was proved yet, a recent study revealed an epidemiological association between chronic periodontitis and erectile dysfunction.

Causes

Periodontitis is an inflammation of the periodontium, i.e., the tissues that support the teeth. The periodontium consists of four tissues:

- gingiva, or gum tissue;
- cementum, or outer layer of the roots of teeth;
- alveolar bone, or the bony sockets into which the teeth are anchored;
- periodontal ligaments (PDLs), which are the connective tissue fibres that run between the cementum and the alveolar bone.

The primary etiology (cause) of gingivitis is poor oral hygiene which leads to the accumulation of a mycotic and bacterial matrix at the gum line, called dental plaque. Other contributors are poor nutrition and underlying medical issues such as diabetes. New finger nick tests have been approved by the Food and Drug Administration in the US, and are being used in dental offices to identify and screen patients for possible contributory causes of gum disease such as diabetes.

In some people, gingivitis progresses to periodontitis –- with the destruction of the gingival fibres, the gum tissues separate from the tooth and deepened sulcus, called a periodontal pocket. Subgingival microorganism (those that exist under the gum line) colonise the periodontal pockets and cause further inflammation in the gum tissues and progressive bone loss. Examples of secondary etiology are those things that, by definition, cause microbic plaque accumulation, such as restoration overhangs and root proximity.

Smoking is another factor that increases the occurrence of periodontitis, directly or indirectly, and may interfere with or adversely affect its treatment.

Ehlers-Danlos Syndrome is a periodontitis risk factor.

If left undisturbed, microbic plaque calcifies to form calculus, which is commonly called tartar. Calculus above and below the gum line must be removed completely by the dental hygienist or dentist to treat gingivitis and periodontitis. Although the primary cause of both gingivitis and periodontitis is the microbic plaque that adheres to the tooth surface, there are many other modifying factors. A very strong risk factor is one's genetic susceptibility. Several conditions and diseases, including Down syndrome, diabetes, and other diseases that affect one's resistance to infection also increase susceptibility to periodontitis.

Another factor that makes periodontitis a difficult disease to study is that human host response can also affect the alveolar bone resorption. Host response to the bacterial-mycotic insult is mainly determined by genetics; however, immune development may play some role in susceptibility.

According to some researches periodontitis may be associated with higher stress.

Prevention

Daily oral hygiene measures to prevent periodontal disease include:

Brushing properly on a regular basis (at least twice daily), with the patient attempting to direct the toothbrush bristles underneath the gum-line, to help disrupt the bacterial-mycotic growth and formation of subgingival plaque.

Flossing daily and using interdental brushes (if there is a sufficiently large space between teeth), as well as cleaning behind the last tooth, the third molar, in each quarter.

Using an antiseptic mouthwash. Chlorhexidine gluconate based mouthwash in combination with careful oral hygiene may cure gingivitis, although they cannot reverse any attachment loss due to periodontitis.

Using a 'soft' tooth brush to prevent damage to tooth enamel and sensitive gums.

Using periodontal trays to maintain dentist-prescribed medications at the source of the disease. The use of trays allows the medication to stay in place long enough to penetrate the biofilms where the microorganism are found.

Regular dental check-ups and professional teeth cleaning as required. Dental check-ups serve to monitor the person's oral hygiene methods and levels of attachment around teeth, identify any early signs of periodontitis, and monitor response to treatment.

Typically dental hygienists (or dentists) use special instruments to clean (debride) teeth below the gumline and disrupt any plaque growing below the gumline. This is a standard treatment to prevent any further progress of established periodontitis. Studies show that after such a professional cleaning (periodontal debridement), microbic plaque tend to grow back to pre-cleaning levels after about 3–4 months. However, it is advocated that the interval between dental check-ups should be determined specifically for each patient between every 3 to 12 months.

Nonetheless, the continued stabilisation of a patient's periodontal state depends largely, if not primarily, on the patient's oral hygiene at home as well as on the go. Without daily oral hygiene, periodontal disease will not be overcome, especially if the patient has a history of extensive periodontal disease.

Periodontal disease and tooth loss are associated with an increased risk of cancer.

A contributing cause may be low selenium in the diet: "Results showed that selenium has the strongest association with gum disease, with low levels increasing the risk by 13 fold."

Management

The cornerstone of successful periodontal treatment starts with establishing excellent oral hygiene. This includes twice daily brushing with daily flossing. Also the use of an interdental brush (called a Proxi-brush) is helpful if space between the teeth allows. For smaller spaces a product called "Soft Picks" are an excellent manual cleaning device. Persons with dexterity problems such as arthritis may find oral hygiene to be difficult and may require more frequent professional care and/or the use of a powered tooth brush. Persons with periodontitis must realise that it is a chronic inflammatory disease and a lifelong regimen of excellent hygiene and professional maintenance care with a dentist/hygienist or periodontist is required to maintain affected teeth.

Initial Therapy

Removal of microbic plaque and calculus is necessary to establish periodontal health. The first step in the treatment of periodontitis involves nonsurgical cleaning below the gumline with a procedure called scaling and debridement. In the past, Root Planing was used (removal of cemental layer as well as calculus). This procedure involves use of specialised curettes to mechanically remove plaque and calculus from below the gumline, and may require multiple visits and local anesthesia to adequately complete. In addition to initial scaling and root planing, it may also be necessary to adjust the occlusion (bite) to prevent excessive force on teeth that have reduced bone support. Also it may be necessary to complete any other dental needs such as replacement of rough, plaque retentive restorations, closure of open contacts between teeth, and any other requirements diagnosed at the initial evaluation.

Reevaluation

Multiple clinical studies have shown that nonsurgical scaling and root planing is usually successful if the periodontal pockets are shallower than 4–5 mm. It is necessary for the dentist or hygienist to perform a reevaluation 4–6 weeks after the initial scaling and root planing, to determine if the patient's oral hygiene has improved and inflammation has regressed. Probing should be avoided at 4–6 weeks, and an analysis by gingival index should determine the presence or absence of inflammation.

Three monthly reevaluation of periodontal therapy should involve periodontal charting as a better indication of the success of treatment, and to see if other courses of treatment can be identified. Pocket depths of greater than 5-6 mm which remain after initial therapy, with bleeding upon probing, indicate continued active disease and will very likely lead to further bone loss over time. This is especially true in molar tooth sites where furcations (areas between the roots) have been exposed.

Surgery

If nonsurgical therapy is found to have been unsuccessful in managing signs of disease activity, periodontal surgery may be needed to stop progressive bone loss and regenerate lost bone where possible. There are many surgical approaches used in treatment of advanced periodontitis, including open flap debridement, osseous surgery, as well as guided tissue regeneration and bone grafting. The goal of periodontal surgery is access for definitive calculus removal and surgical management of bony irregularities which have resulted from the disease process to reduce pockets as much as possible. Long-term studies have shown that in moderate to advanced periodontitis, surgically treated cases often have less further breakdown over time and when coupled with a regular post-treatment maintenance regimen are successful in nearly halting tooth loss in nearly 85% of patients.

Maintenance

Once successful periodontal treatment has been completed, with or without surgery, an ongoing regimen of "periodontal maintenance" is required. This involves regular checkups and detailed cleanings every three months to prevent re-population of periodontitis-causing microorganism, and to closely monitor affected teeth so that early treatment can be rendered if disease recurs. Usually periodontal disease exists due to poor plaque control, therefore if the brushing techniques are not modified, a periodontal recurrence is probable.

Alternative Treatments

Periodontitis has an inescapable relationship with subgingival calculus (tartar). The first step in any procedure is to eliminate calculus under the gum line, as it houses destructive anaerobic microorganisms that consume bone, gum and cementum (connective tissue) for food.

Most alternative "at-home" gum disease treatments involve injecting antimicrobial solutions, such as hydrogen peroxide, into periodontal pockets via slender applicators or oral irrigators. This process disrupts anaerobic microorganism colonies and is effective at reducing infections and inflammation when used daily. A number of potions and elixirs that are functionally equivalent to hydrogen peroxide are commercially available but at substantially higher cost. However, such treatments do not address calculus formations, and so are short-lived, as anaerobic microorganism colonies quickly regenerate in and around calculus.

In a new field of study, calculus formations are addressed on a more fundamental level. At the heart of the formation of subgingival calculus, growing plaque formations starve out the lowest members of the community, which calcify into calcium phosphate salts of the same shape and size of the original, organic bacilli. Calcium phosphate salts (unlike calcium phosphate; the primary component in teeth) are ionic and adhere to tooth surfaces via electrostatic attraction. Smaller, free-floating calcium phosphate salt particles are equally attracted to the same areas, as are additional calcified microorganism, growing calculus formations as unorganised, yet strong, "brick and mortar" matrices. The microscopic voids in calculus formations house new anaerobic microorganism, as does the top "diseased layer".

Because the root cause of subgingival calculus development is ionic attraction, it was hypothesized that the introduction of oppositely charged particles around the formations may chelate calcium phosphate salt components away from the matrix, thus reducing the size of subgingival calculus formations. To accomplish this, a sequestering agent solution consisting partly of sodium tripolyphosphate (STPP) and sodium fluoride (charge -1) was tested on a patient with burnished and new subgingival calculus at a depth of 6 mm. The patient delivered the solution using an oral irrigator, once a day, for 60 days. The results were the successful elimination of all calculus formations studied. This test was conducted using a subgingival endoscopic camera (perioscope) by an independent periodontist.

The promise of this new, alternative treatment is to keep subgingival calculus at bay, in concert with traditional periodontal treatments. In this way, periodontitis may be controlled by the patient, and complete restoration of dental health can be a collaborative effort between the patient and the dental professional.

Additionally, Periodontitis can be treated in a noninvasive manner by means of Periostat (subantimicrobial dose of doxycycline), an FDA-approved, orally-administered drug that has been shown to reduce bone loss. Its mechanism of action in part involves inhibition of Matrix metalloproteinases (such as collagenase), which degrade the extracellular matrix under inflammatory conditions. This ultimately can lead to reduction of aveolar bone-loss in patients with periodontal disease (as well as patients without periodontitis).

Prognosis

Dentists and dental hygienists measure periodontal disease using a device called a periodontal probe. This is a thin "measuring stick" that is gently placed into the space between the gums and the teeth, and slipped below the gum-line. If the probe can slip more than 3 millimetres below the gum-line, the patient is said to have a gingival pocket if no migration of the epithelial attachment has occurred or a periodontal pocket if apical migration has occurred. This is somewhat of a misnomer, as any depth is in essence a pocket, which in turn is defined by its depth, i.e., a 2 mm pocket or a 6 mm pocket.

However, it is generally accepted that pockets are self-cleansable (at home, by the patient, with a toothbrush) if they are 3 mm or less in depth. This is important because if there is a pocket which is deeper than 3 mm around the tooth, at-home care will not be sufficient to cleanse the pocket, and professional care should be sought. When the pocket depths reach 6 and 7 mm in depth, the hand instruments and cavitrons used by the dental professionals may not reach deeply enough into the pocket to clean out the microbic plaque that cause gingival inflammation. In such a situation the bone or the gums around that tooth should be surgically altered or it will always have inflammation which will likely result in more bone loss around that tooth. An additional way to stop the inflammation would be for the patient to receive subgingival antibiotics (such as minocycline) or undergo some form of gingival surgery to access the depths of the pockets and perhaps even change the pocket depths so that they become 3 mm or less in depth and can once again be properly cleaned by the patient at home with his or her toothbrush.

If a patient has 7 mm or deeper pockets around their teeth, then they would likely risk eventual tooth loss over the years. If this periodontal condition is not identified and the patient remains unaware of the progressive nature of the disease then, years later, they may be surprised that some teeth will gradually become loose and may need to be extracted, sometimes due to a severe infection or even pain.

According to the Sri Lankan tea labourer study, in the absence of any oral hygiene activity, approximately 10% will suffer from severe periodontal disease with rapid loss of attachment (>2 mm/ year). 80% will suffer from moderate loss (1–2 mm/year) and the remaining 10% will not suffer any loss.

Epidemiology

Periodontitis is very common, and is widely regarded as the second most common disease worldwide, after dental decay, and in the United States has a prevalence of 30–50% of the population, but only about 10% have severe forms.

Like other conditions that are intimately related to access to hygiene and basic medical monitoring and care, periodontitis tends to be more common in economically disadvantaged populations or regions. Its occurrence decreases with higher standard of living. In Israeli population, individuals of Yemenite, North-African, South Asian, or Mediterranean origin have higher prevalence of periodontal disease than individuals from European descent.

Presumably, individuals living in East Asia (e.g. Japan, South Korea and Taiwan) have the lowest incident of periodontal disease in the world.

In other Animals

Periodontal disease is the most common disease found in dogs and affects more than 80% of dogs aged three years or older. The prevalence of periodontal disease in dogs increases with age but decreases with increasing body weight; i.e., toy and miniature breeds are more severely affected. Systemic disease may develop because the gums are very vascular (have a good blood supply). The blood stream carries these anaerobic microorganisms, and they are filtered out by the kidneys and liver, where they may colonise and create microabscesses. The microorganisms travelling through the blood may also attach to the heart valves, causing vegetative endocarditis (infected heart valves). Additional diseases that may result from periodontitis includes chronic bronchitis and pulmonary fibrosis.

Candidiasis

Candidiasis or thrush is a fungal infection (mycosis) of any of the *Candida* species (all yeasts), of which *Candida albicans* is the most common. Also commonly referred to as a yeast infection, candidiasis is also technically known as candidosis, moniliasis, and oidiomycosis.

Candidiasis encompasses infections that range from superficial, such as oral thrush and vaginitis, to systemic and potentially life-threatening diseases. *Candida* infections of the latter category are also referred to as candidemia and are usually confined to severely immunocompromised persons, such as cancer, transplant, and AIDS patients as well as non-trauma emergency surgery patients.

Superficial infections of skin and mucosal membranes by *Candida* causing local inflammation and discomfort are common in many human populations. While clearly attributable to the presence of the opportunistic pathogens of the genus *Candida*, candidiasis describes a number of different disease syndromes that often differ in their causes and outcomes.

Classification

Candidiasis may be divided into the following types:
- Oral candidiasis (Thrush)
- Perlèche (Angular cheilitis)
- Candidal vulvovaginitis (vaginal yeast infection)
- Candidal intertrigo
- Diaper candidiasis
- Congenital cutaneous candidiasis
- Perianal candidiasis
- Candidal paronychia
- Erosio interdigitalis blastomycetica

- Chronic mucocutaneous candidiasis
- Systemic candidiasis
- Candidid
- Antibiotic candidiasis (Iatrogenic candidiasis).

Signs and Symptoms

Most candidial infections are treatable and result in minimal complications such as redness, itching and discomfort, though complication may be severe or fatal if left untreated in certain populations. In immunocompetent persons, candidiasis is usually a very localised infection of the skin or mucosal membranes, including the oral cavity (thrush), the pharynx or esophagus, the gastrointestinal tract, the urinary bladder, or the genitalia (vagina, penis).

Candidiasis is a very common cause of vaginal irritation, or vaginitis, and can also occur on the male genitals. In immunocompromised patients, *Candida* infections can affect the esophagus with the potential of becoming systemic, causing a much more serious condition, a fungemia called candidemia.

Thrush is commonly seen in infants. It is not considered abnormal in infants unless it lasts longer than a couple of weeks. Children, mostly between the ages of three and nine years of age, can be affected by chronic mouth yeast infections, normally seen around the mouth as white patches. However, this is not a common condition.

Symptoms of candidiasis may vary depending on the area affected. Infection of the vagina or vulva may cause severe itching, burning, soreness, irritation, and a whitish or whitish-gray cottage cheese-like discharge, often with a curd-like appearance. These symptoms are also present in the more common bacterial vaginosis. In a 2002 study published in the *Journal of Obstetrics and Gynecology*, only 33 percent of women who were self-treating for a yeast infection actually had a yeast infection, while most had either bacterial vaginosis or a mixed-type infection. Symptoms of infection of the male genitalia include red patchy sores near the head of the penis or on the foreskin, severe itching, or a burning sensation. Candidiasis of the penis can also have a white discharge, although uncommon.

Causes

Candida yeasts are commonly present in humans, and their growth is normally limited by the human immune system and by other microorganisms, such as bacteria occupying the same locations (niches) in the human body.

C. albicans was isolated from the vaginas of 19% of apparently healthy women, i.e., those that experienced few or no symptoms of infection. External use of detergents or douches or internal disturbances (hormonal or physiological) can perturb the normal vaginal flora, consisting of lactic acid bacteria, such as lactobacilli, and result in an overgrowth of *Candida* cells causing symptoms of infection, such as local inflammation.

Pregnancy and the use of oral contraceptives have been reported as risk factors, while the roles of engaging in vaginal sex immediately and without cleansing after anal sex and using lubricants containing glycerin remain controversial. Diabetes mellitus and the use of antibacterial antibiotics are also linked to an increased incidence of yeast infections. Diet high in carbohydrates has been found to affect rates of oral candidiases, and hormone replacement therapy and infertility treatments may also be predisposing factors. Wearing wet swimwear for long periods of time is also believed to be a risk factor.

A weakened or undeveloped immune system or metabolic illnesses such as diabetes are significant predisposing factors of candidiasis. Diseases or conditions linked to candidiasis include HIV/AIDS, mononucleosis, cancer treatments, steroids, stress, and nutrient deficiency.

Almost 15% of people with weakened immune systems develop a systemic illness caused by *Candida* species. In extreme cases, these superficial infections of the skin or mucous membranes may enter into the bloodstream and cause systemic *Candida* infections.

In penile candidiasis, the causes include sexual intercourse with an infected individual, low immunity, antibiotics, and diabetes. Male genital yeast infection is less common, and incidence of infection is only a fraction of that in women; however, yeast infection on the penis from direct contact via sexual intercourse with an infected partner is not uncommon.

Candida species are frequently part of the human body's normal oral and intestinal flora. Treatment with antibiotics can lead to eliminating the yeast's natural competitors for resources, and increase the severity of the condition. Higher prevalence of colonisation of *C. albicans* was reported in young individuals with tongue piercing, in comparison to non-tongue-pierced matched individuals. In the western hemisphere approximately 75% of females are affected at some time in their life.

Diagnosis

Diagnosis of a yeast infection is done either via microscopic examination or culturing.

For identification by light microscopy, a scraping or swab of the affected area is placed on a microscope slide. A single drop of 10% potassium hydroxide (KOH) solution is then added to the specimen. The KOH dissolves the skin cells but leaves the *Candida* cells intact, permitting visualisation of pseudohyphae and budding yeast cells typical of many *Candida* species.

For the culturing method, a sterile swab is rubbed on the infected skin surface. The swab is then streaked on a culture medium. The culture is incubated at 37 °C for several days, to allow development of yeast or bacterial colonies. The characteristics (such as morphology and colour) of the colonies may allow initial diagnosis of the organism that is causing disease symptoms.

Treatment

In clinical settings, candidiasis is commonly treated with antimycotics—the antifungal drugs commonly used to treat candidiasis are topical clotrimazole, topical nystatin, fluconazole, and topical ketoconazole.

For example, a one-time dose of fluconazole (150 mg tablet taken orally) has been reported as being 90% effective in treating a vaginal yeast infection. This dose is only effective for vaginal yeast infections, and other types of yeast infections may require different dosing. In severe infections amphotericin B, caspofungin, or voriconazole may be used.

Local treatment may include vaginal suppositories or medicated douches. Gentian violet can be used for breastfeeding thrush, but when used in large quantities it can cause mouth and throat ulcerations in nursing babies, and has been linked to mouth cancer in humans and to cancer in the digestive tract of other animals.

Chlorhexidine gluconate oral rinse is not recommended to treat candidiasis but is effective as prophylaxis; chlorine dioxide rinse was found to have similar in vitro effectiveness against *candida*.

C. albicans can develop resistance to antimycotic drugs. Recurring infections may be treatable with other antifungal drugs, but resistance to these alternative agents may also develop.

History

The genus *Candida* and species *C. albicans* was described by botanist Christine Marie Berkhout in her doctoral thesis at the University of Utrecht in 1923. Over the years, the classification of the genera and species has evolved. Obsolete names for this genus include *Mycotorula* and *Torulopsis*. The species has also been known in the past as *Monilia albicans* and *Oidium albicans*. The current classification is *nomen conservandum*, which means the name is authorised for use by the International Botanical Congress (IBC).

The genus *Candida* includes about 150 different species, however, only a few are known to cause human infections: *C. albicans* is the most significant pathogenic species. Other *Candida* species pathogenic in humans include *C. tropicalis*, *C. glabrata*, *C. krusei*, *C. parapsilosis*, *C. dubliniensis*, and *C. lusitaniae*.

Society and Culture

Some alternative medicine proponents postulate a widespread occurrence of systemic candidiasis (or candida hypersensitivity syndrome, yeast allergy, or gastrointestinal candida overgrowth). The view was most widely promoted in a book published by Dr. William Crook, which hypothesized that a variety of common symptoms such as fatigue, PMS, sexual dysfunction, asthma, psoriasis, digestive and urinary problems, multiple sclerosis, and muscle pain, could be caused by subclinical infections of *Candida albicans*. Crook suggested a variety of remedies to treat these symptoms, ranging from dietary modification, prescription antifungals, to colonic irrigation. With the exception of the few dietary studies in the urinary tract infection section, conventional medicine has not used most of these alternatives, since there is limited scientific evidence to prove either their effectiveness, or that subclinical systemic candidiasis is a viable diagnosis.

Coccidia

Coccidia is a subclass of microscopic, spore-forming, single-celled obligate parasites belonging to the apicomplexan class Conoidasida. Coccidian parasites infect the intestinal tracts of animals, and are the largest group of apicomplexan protozoa.

Coccidia are obligate, intracellular parasites, which means that they must live and reproduce within an animal cell.

They form a subclass within the Conoidasida and are divided into four orders distinguished by the presence or absence of various asexual and sexual stages.

Taxonomy

- Order *Adelidea* Ledger 1911
- Order *Agamococcidiida* Levine 1979
- Order *Coccidiida* Leukart 1879
- Order *Protococcidiida* Cheissin 1956

The order Coccidia is divided into two groups. The ûrst group (suborder Adeleorina) comprises coccidia of invertebrates and the coccidia that alternate between blood-sucking invertebrates and various vertebrates; this group includes *Hemogregarina* and *Hepatozoon*.

The second group (suborder Eimeriorina) comprises coccidia of vertebrates as well as cyst-forming coccidia, including *Toxoplasma* and *Sarcocystis*. The fundamental difference between these two groups lies in their sexual development: syzygy for Adeleorina and independent gametes for Eimeriorina.

Coccidiosis

Coccidiosis is the disease caused by coccidian infection. Coccidiosis is a parasitic disease of the intestinal tract of animals, caused by coccidian protozoa. The disease spreads from one animal to another by contact with infected feces or ingestion of infected tissue. Diarrhea, which may become bloody in severe cases, is the primary symptom. Most animals infected with coccidia are asymptomatic; however, young or immuno-compromised animals may suffer severe symptoms, including death.

While coccidian organisms can infect a wide variety of animals, including humans, birds, and livestock, they are usually species-specific. One well-known exception is toxoplasmosis, caused by *Toxoplasma gondii*.

People often first encounter coccidia when they acquire a young puppy or kitten who is infected. The infectious organisms are canine/feline-specific and are not contagious to humans (compare to zoonotic diseases).

Coccidia in Dogs

Young puppies are frequently infected with coccidia and often develop active Coccidiosis—even puppies obtained from diligent professional breeders. Infected puppies almost always have received the parasite from their mother's feces. Typically, healthy adult animals shedding the parasite's oocysts in their feces will be asymptomatic because of their developed immune systems. However, undeveloped immune systems make puppies more susceptible. Further, stressors such as new owners, travel, weather changes, and unsanitary conditions are believed to activate infections in susceptible animals.

Symptoms in young dogs are universal: at some point around 2–3 months of age, an infected dog develops persistently loose stools. This diarrhea proceeds to stool containing liquid, thick mucus, and light coloured faecal matter. As the infection progresses, spots of blood may become apparent in the stool, and sudden bowel movements may surprise both dog and owner alike. Other symptoms may include poor appetite, vomiting, dehydration, and sometimes death. Coccidia infection is so common that any pup under 4 months old with these symptoms can almost surely be assumed to have coccidiosis.

Fortunately, the treatment is inexpensive, extremely effective, and routine. A veterinarian can easily diagnose the disease through low-powered microscopic examination of an affected dog's feces, which usually will be replete with oocysts. One of many easily administered and inexpensive drugs will be prescribed, and, in the course of just a few days, an infection will be eliminated or perhaps reduced to such a level that the dog's immune system can make its own progress against the infection. Even when an infection has progressed sufficiently that blood is present in feces, permanent damage to the gastrointestinal system is rare, and the dog will most likely make a complete recovery without long-lasting negative effects.

If one dog of a litter has coccidiosis, then most certainly all dogs at a breeder's kennels have active coccidia infections. Breeders should be notified if a newly-acquired pup is discovered to be infected with coccidia. Breeders can take steps to eradicate the organism from their kennels, including applying medications in bulk to an entire facility.

Genera and Species that Cause Coccidiosis

Genus *Isospora* is the most common cause of intestinal coccidiosis in dogs and cats and is usually what is meant by coccidiosis. Species of *Isospora* are species specific, meaning they only infect one type of species. Species that infect dogs include *I. canis*, *I. ohioensis*, *I. burrowsi*, and *I. neorivolta*. Species that infect cats include *I. felis* and *I. rivolta*. The most common symptom is diarrhea. sulfonamides are the most common treatment.

Genus *Cryptosporidium* contains two species known to cause cryptosporidiosis, *C. parvum* and *C. muris*. Cattle are most commonly affected by *Cryptosporidium*, and their feces are often assumed to be a source of infection for other mammals including humans. Recent genetic analyses of *Cryptosporidium* in humans have identified *Cryptosporidium hominis* as a new species specific for humans. Infection occurs most commonly in individuals that are immunocompromised, e.g. dogs with canine distemper, cats with feline leukemia virus infection, and humans with AIDS. Very young puppies and kittens can also become infected with *Cryptosporidium*, but the infection is usually eliminated without treatment.

Genus *Hammondia* is transmitted by ingestion of cysts found in the tissue of grasing animals and rodents. Dogs and cats are the definitive hosts, with the species H. heydorni infecting dogs and the species H. hammondi and H. pardalis infecting cats. Hammondia usually does not cause disease.

Genus *Besnoitia* infect cats that ingest cysts found in the tissue of rodents and opossum, but usually does not cause disease.

Genus *Sarcocystis* infect carnivores that ingest cysts from various intermediate hosts. It is possible for *Sarcocystis* to cause disease in dogs and cats.

Genus *Toxoplasma* has one important species, *Toxoplasma gondii*. Cats are the definitive host, but all mammals and some fish, reptiles, and amphibians can be intermediate hosts. Therefore, only cat feces will hold infective oocysts, but infection through ingestion of cysts can occur with the tissue of any intermediate host. Toxoplasmosis occurs in humans usually as low-grade fever or muscle pain for a few days. A normal immune system will suppress the infection but the tissue cysts will persist in that animal or human for years or the rest of its life. In immunocompromised individuals, those dormant cysts can be reactivated and cause many lesions in the brain, heart, lungs, eyes, etc. Without a competent immune system, the animal or human will most likely die from the infection. For pregnant women, the fetus is at risk if the pregnant woman becomes infected for the first time during pregnancy. If the woman had been infected during childhood or adolescence, she will have an immunity that will protect her developing fetus during pregnancy.

The most important misconception about the transmission of toxoplasmosis comes from statements like 'ingestion of raw or undercooked meat, or cat feces.' Kitchen hygiene is much more important because people do tend to taste marinades or sauces before being cooked, or chop meat then vegetables without properly cleaning the knife and cutting board. Many physicians mistakenly put panic in their pregnant clients and advise them to get rid of their cat without really warning them of the likely sources of infection. Adult cats are very unlikely to shed infective oocysts. Symptoms in cats include fever, weight loss, diarrhea, vomiting, uveitis, and central nervous system signs. Disease in dogs includes a rapidly progressive form seen in dogs also infected with distemper, and a neurological form causing paralysis, tremors, and seizures. Dogs and cats are usually treated with clindamycin.

Genus *Neospora* has one important species, *Neospora caninum*, that affects dogs in a manner similar to toxoplasmosis. Neosporosis is difficult to treat.

Genus *Hepatozoon* contains one species that causes hepatozoonosis in dogs and cats, *Hepatozoon canis*. Animals become infected by ingesting an infected *Rhipicephalus sanguineus*, also known as the brown dog tick. Symptoms include fever, weight loss, and pain of the spine and limbs.

The most common medications used to treat coccidian infections are in the sulphonamide family. Although unusual, sulphonamides can damage the tear glands in some dogs, causing *keratoconjunctivitis sicca*, or "dry eye", which may have a life-long impact. Some veterinarians recommend measuring tear production prior to sulphonamide administration, and at various intervals after administration. Other veterinarians will simply avoid using sulphonamides, instead choosing another product effective against coccidia.

Left untreated, the infection may clear of its own accord, or in some cases may continue to ravage an animal and cause permanent damage or, occasionally, death.

Cryptosporidiosis

Cryptosporidiosis, also known as crypto, is a parasitic disease caused by *Cryptosporidium*, a protozoan parasite in the phylum Apicomplexa. It affects the intestines of mammals and is typically an acute short-term infection. It is spread through the faecal-oral route, often through contaminated water; the main symptom is self-limiting diarrhea in people with intact immune systems. In immunocompromised individuals, such as AIDS patients, the symptoms are particularly severe and often fatal. *Cryptosporidium* is the organism most commonly isolated in HIV positive patients presenting with diarrhea. Treatment is symptomatic, with fluid rehydration, electrolyte correction and management of any pain. Despite not being identified until 1976, it is one of the most common waterborne diseases and is found worldwide. The parasite is transmitted by environmentally hardy microbial cysts (oocysts) that, once ingested, exist in the small intestine and result in an infection of intestinal epithelial tissue.

History

The organism was first described in 1907 by Tyzzer, who recognised it was a coccidian.

General Characteristics of Cryptosporidium

Cryptosporidium is a protozoan pathogen of the Phylum Apicomplexa and causes a diarrheal illness called cryptosporidiosis. Other apicomplexan pathogens include the malaria parasite *Plasmodium*, and *Toxoplasma*, the causative agent of toxoplasmosis. Unlike *Plasmodium*, which transmits via a mosquito vector, *Cryptosporidium* does not require an insect vector and is capable of completing its life cycle within a single host, resulting in microbial cyst stages which are excreted in feces and are capable of transmission to a new host. However, studies show that synanthropic filth flies may be involved in the transmission of human and animal cryptosporidiosis.

The pattern of Cryptosporidium life cycle fits well that of other intestinal homogeneous coccidian genera of the suborder *Eimeriina*: macro and microgamonts develop independently; a microgamont gives rise to numerous male gametes; and oocysts serving for parasites' spreading in the environment.

Electron microscopic studies made from the 1970s have shown the intracellular, although extracytoplasmic localisation of

Cryptosporidium species. These Species Possess a Number of Unusual features:

- an endogenous phase of development in microvilli of epithelial surfaces
- two morphofunctional types of oocysts
- the smallest number of sporozoites per oocyst
- a multi-membraneous "feeder" organelle.

DNA studies suggest a relationship with the gregarines rather than the coccidia. The taxonomic position of this group has not yet been finally agreed upon.

The genome of *Cryptosporidium parvum* was sequenced in 2004 and was found to be unusual amongst Eukaryotes in that the mitochondria seem not to contain DNA. A closely related species, *C. hominis*, also has its genome sequence available. CryptoDB.org is a NIH-funded database that provides access to the *Cryptosporidium* genomics data sets.

A number of *Cryptosporidium* infect mammals. In humans, the main causes of disease are *C. parvum* and *C. hominis* (previously *C. parvum* genotype 1). *C. canis*, *C. felis*, *C. meleagridis*, and *C. muris* can also cause disease in humans.

Cryptosporidiosis is typically an acute short-term infection but can become severe and non-resolving in children and immunocompromised individuals. In humans, it remains in the lower intestine and may remain for up to five weeks. The parasite is transmitted by environmentally hardy microbial cysts (oocysts) that, once ingested, exist in the small intestine and result in an infection of intestinal epithelial tissue.

Infection is through contaminated material such as earth, water, uncooked or cross-contaminated food that has been in contact with the feces of an infected individual or animal. Contact must then be transferred to the mouth and swallowed. It is especially prevalent amongst those in regular contact with bodies of fresh water including recreational water such as swimming pools. Other potential sources include insufficiently treated water supplies, contaminated food, or exposure to feces. The high resistance of *Cryptosporidium* oocysts to disinfectants such as chlorine bleach enables them to survive for long periods and still remain infective. Some outbreaks have happened in day care related to diaper changes.

Symptoms

Symptoms appear from two to ten days after infection, with an average of 7 days, and last for up to two weeks, or in some cases, up to one month. There are 3 possible forms of the illness in immunocompetent people. The disease can be asymptomatic or cause acute diarrhea or persistent diarrhea that can last for a few weeks. Diarrhea is usually watery with mucus. It is very rare to find blood or leukocytes in the diarrhea. As well as watery diarrhea, there is often stomach pains or cramps and a low fever. Other symptoms include nausea, vomiting, malabsorption and dehydration. The individuals who are asymptomatic (have no symptoms) are nevertheless infective, and thus can pass on the infection to others. Even after symptoms have finally subsided an individual is still infective for some weeks.

Severe diseases, including pancreatitis, can occur.

Immunocompromised people, as well as very young or very old people, can develop a more severe form of cryptosporidiosis. There are 4 clinical presentations for patients with AIDS. 4% have no symptoms, 29% have a transient infection, 60% have chronic diarrhea, and 8% have a severe, cholera-like infection. With transient infections diarrhea ends within 2 months and Cryptosporidium is no longer found in the feces. Chronic diarrhea is diarrhea that lasts for 2 or more months. The most severe form results in the patients excreting at least 2 litres of watery diarrhea per day. They can lose up to 25 litres per day. AIDS patients can have up to 10 stools per day. They experience severe malabsorption and can have 10% weight loss. Many of them never completely eliminate *Cryptosporidium* from their bodies.

When Cryptosporidium spreads beyond the intestine, as it can predominantly in patients with AIDS, it can reach the lungs, middle ear, pancreas, and stomach. Thus, one symptom is pain in the right upper quadrant. The parasite can infect the biliary tract, causing biliary cryptosporidiosis. This can result in cholecystitis and cholangitis.

Life Cycle

Cryptosporidium has a spore phase (oocyst) and in this state it can survive for lengthy periods outside a host. It can also resist many common disinfectants, notably chlorine-based disinfectants.

The life cycle of *Cryptosporidium parvum* consists of an asexual stage and a sexual stage. After being ingested, the oocysts excyst in the small intestine. They release sporozoites that attach to the microvilli of the epithelial cells of the small intestine. From there they become trophozoites that reproduce asexually by multiple fission, a process known as schizogony. The trophozoites develop into Type 1 meronts that contain 8 daughter cells. These daughter cells are Type 1 merozoites, which get released by the meronts. Some of these merozoites can cause autoinfection by attaching to epithelial cells. Others of these merozoites become Type II meronts, which contain 4 Type II merozoites. These merozoites get released and they attach to the epithelial cells. From there they become either macrogamonts or microgamonts. These are the female and male sexual forms, respectively. This stage, when sexual forms arise, is called gametogony. Zygotes are formed by microgametes from the microgamont penetrating the macrogamonts. The zygotes develop into oocysts of two types. 20% of oocysts have thin walls and so can reinfect the host by rupturing and releasing sporozoites that start the process over again. The thick-walled oocysts are excreted into the environment. The oocysts are mature and infective upon being excreted. They can survive in the environment for months.

Pathogenesis

The oocysts are ovoid or spherical and measure 5 to 6 micrometres across. When in flotation preparations they appear highly refractile. The oocysts contains up to 4 sporozoites that are bow-shaped.

As few as 2 to 10 oocysts can initiate an infection. The parasite is located in the brush border of the epithelial cells of the small intestine. They are mainly located in the jejunum. When the sporozoites attach the epithelial cells' membrane envelops them. Thus, they are "intracellular but extracytoplasmic". The parasite can cause damage to the microvilli where it attaches. The infected human excretes the most oocysts during the first week. Oocysts can be excreted for weeks after the diarrhea subsides.

The immune system reduces the formation of Type 1 merozoites as well as the number of thin-walled oocysts. This helps prevent autoinfection. B cells do not help with the initial response or the fight to eliminate the parasite.

Diagnostic Tests

There are many diagnostic tests for *Cryptosporidium*. They include microscopy, staining, and detection of antibodies. Microscopy can help identify oocysts in faecal matter. To increase the chance of finding the oocysts, the diagnostician should inspect at least 3 stool samples. There are several techniques to concentrate either the stool sample or the oocysts. The modified formalin-ethyl acetate (FEA) concentration method concentrates the stool. Both the modified zinc sulfate centrifugal flotation technique and the Sheather's sugar flotation procedure can concentrate the oocysts by causing them to float. Another form of microscopy is fluorescent microscopy done by staining with auramine.

Other staining techniques include acid-fast staining, which will stain the oocysts red. One type of acid-fast stain is the Kinyoun technique. Giemsa staining can also be performed. Part of the small intestine can be stained with hematoxylin and eosin (H & E), which will show oocysts attached to the epithelial cells.

Detecting antigens is yet another way to diagnose the disease. This can be done with direct fluorescent antibody (DFA) techniques. It can also be achieved through indirect immunofluorescence assay. Enzyme-Linked ImmunoSorbent Assay (ELISA) also detects antigens.

Polymerase chain reaction (PCR) is another way to diagnose cryptosporidiosis. It can even identify the specific species of *Cryptosporidium*. If the patient is thought to have biliary cryptosporidiosis, then an appropriate diagnostic technique is ultrasonography. If that returns normal results, the next step would be to perform endoscopic retrograde cholangiopancreatography.

Treatment

There is no reliable treatment for cryptosporidium enteritis; certain agents such as paromomycin, atovaquone, nitazoxanide, and azithromycin are sometimes used, but they usually have only temporary effects.

Treatment is primarily supportive. Fluids need to be replaced orally. A lactose-free diet should be taken as tolerated. In rare situations, intravenous fluids may be required. Antibiotics are not usually helpful, and are primarily reserved for persons with severe disease and a weak immune system. Sometimes relapses happen.

In the Immunocompetent

The majority of immunocompetent individuals suffer a short (less than 2 weeks) self-limiting course that requires supportive care with rehydration and occasionally antidiarrhoeal medication, and ends with spontaneous recovery. Nitazoxanide is one drug that the US FDA has approved for use in immunocompetent people to combat diarrhea. Spiramycin can help shorten the amount of time oocysts are passed, as well as the duration of diarrhoea in children.

In the Immunocompromised

In immunocompromised individuals, such as AIDS patients, cryptosporidiosis resolves slowly or not at all, and frequently causes a particularly severe and permanent form of watery diarrhea coupled with a greatly decreased ability to absorb key nutrients through the intestinal tract. The result is progressively severe dehydration, electrolyte imbalances, malnutrition, wasting, and eventual death. Spiramycin can help treat diarrhea in patients who are in the early stages of AIDS. The mortality rate for infected AIDS patients is generally based on CD4+ marker counts; patients with CD4+ counts over 180 cells/mm^3 generally recover with supportive hospital care and medication, but in patients with CD4+ counts below 50 cells/mm^3, the effects are usually fatal within three to six months. During the Milwaukee cryptosporidiosis epidemic (the largest of its kind), 73% of AIDS patients with CD4+ counts lower than 50 cells/mm^3 and 36% of those with counts between 50 and 200 cells/mm^3 died within the first year of contracting the infection. In one AIDS patient from Iran, who had pulmonary cryptosporidiosis in addition to intestinal cryptosporidiosis, azithromycin and paromomycin helped to clear the infection.

Currently, the best approach is to improve the immune status in immunodeficient individuals, which causes the diarrhea resolve for itself in most of the cases. Biliar drainage may be needed in case the biliary tract is affected.

Currently, research is being done in molecular-based immunotherapy. For example, synthetic isoflavone derivates have been shown to fight off *Cryptosporidium parvum* in vitro and in a gerbil. Derivates of nitazoxanide, which are synthetic nitro or nonnitrothiazolide compounds.

Treatment of Drinking Water

Many treatment plants that take raw water from rivers, lakes, and reservoirs for public drinking water production use conventional filtration technologies. This involves a series of processes, including coagulation, flocculation, sedimentation, and filtration. Direct filtration, which is typically used to treat water with low particulate levels, includes coagulation and filtration, but not sedimentation. Other common filtration processes, including slow sand filters, diatomaceous earth filters and membranes will remove 99% of *Cryptosporidium*. Membranes and bag and cartridge filters remove *Cryptosporidium* product-specifically.

While *Cryptosporidium* is highly resistant to chlorine disinfection, with high enough concentrations and contact time, *Cryptosporidium* will be inactivated by chlorine dioxide and ozone treatment. The required levels of chlorine generally preclude the use of chlorine disinfection as a reliable method to control *Cryptosporidium* in drinking water. Ultraviolet light treatment at relatively low doses will inactivate *Cryptosporidium*. Water Research Foundation-funded research originally discovered UV's efficacy in inactivating *Cryptosporidium*.

One of the largest challenges in identifying outbreaks is the ability to identify *Cryptosporidium* in the laboratory. Real-time monitoring technology is now able to detect *Cryptosporidium* with online systems, unlike the spot and batch testing methods used in the past.

The most reliable way to decontaminate drinking water which may be contaminated by *Cryptosporidium* is to boil it.

Non-human Examples

The most important zoonotic reservoirs are cattle, sheep and goats. Additionally, in recent years, cryptosporidiosis has plagued many commercial leopard gecko breeders. Several species of the Cryptosporidium family (C. serpentes and others) are involved, and outside of geckos it has been found in monitor lizards, iguanas and tortoises, as well as several snake species.

Exposure Risks

Cryptosporidiosis is found worldwide. It causes 50.8% of water-borne diseases that are attributed to parasites. In developing countries, 8-19% of diarrheal diseases can be attributed to *Cryptosporidium*. Ten percent of the population in developing countries excretes oocysts. In developed countries, the number is lower at 1-3%. The age group most affected is children from 1 to 9 years old.

The following groups have an elevated risk of being exposed to Cryptosporidium:

- People who swim regularly in pools with insufficient sanitation (certain strains of *Cryptosporidium* are chlorine-resistant)
- Child care workers
- Parents of infected children
- People who take care of other people with cryptosporidiosis
- International travellers
- Backpackers, hikers, and campers who drink unfiltered, untreated water
- People, including swimmers, who swallow water from contaminated sources
- People who handle infected cattle
- People exposed to human feces through sexual contact.

Cases of cryptosporidiosis can occur in a city that does not have a contaminated water supply. In a city with clean water, it may be that cases of cryptosporidiosis have different origins. Testing of water, as well as epidemiological study, are necessary to determine the sources of specific infections. Note that *Cryptosporidium* typically does not cause serious illness in healthy people. It may chronically sicken some children, as well as adults who are exposed and immunocompromised. A subset of the immunocompromised population is people with AIDS. Some sexual behaviours can transmit the parasite directly.

Table : Statistics for the United States - number of cases:

Year	Cases
2006	5,936
2007	11,170
2008	7,749

Public Health and Prevention Strategies

In the US the law requires doctors and labs to report cases of cryptosporidiosis to local or state health departments. These departments then report to the Centre for Disease Control and Prevention. The best way to prevent getting and spreading cryptosporidiosis is to have good hygiene and sanitation. An example would be hand-washing. Prevention is through washing hands carefully after going to the bathroom or contacting stool, and before eating. People should avoid contact with animal feces. They should also avoid possibly contaminated food and water. Additionally, people should refrain from engaging in sexual activities that can expose them to feces.

Standard water filtration may not be enough to eliminate *Cryptosporidium*; boiling for at least 1 minute (3 minutes above 6,500 feet (2,000 m) of altitude) will decontaminate it. Heating milk at 71.7 °C for 15 seconds pasteurizes it and can destroy the oocysts' ability to infect. Water can also be made safe by filtering with a filter with pore size not greater than 1 micrometre, or by filters that have been approved for "cyst removal" by the US National Science Foundation (NSF). Bottled drinking water is less likely to contain *Cryptosporidium*, especially if the water is from an underground source.

People who have cryptosporidiosis should not swim in communal areas because the pathogen can reside in the anal and genital areas and be washed off. They should wait until at least two weeks after diarrhea stops before entering public water sources, since oocysts can still be shed for a while. Also, they should stay away from immunosuppressed people. Immunocompromised people should take care to protect themselves from water in lakes and streams. They should also stay away from animal stools and wash their hands after touching animals. To be safe, they should boil or filter their water. They should also wash and cook their vegetables.

Notable Cases

In 1987, 13,000 people in Carrollton, Georgia, became ill with cryptosporidiosis. This was the first report of its spread through a municipal water system that met all state and federal drinking water standards.

In 1993, a waterborne cryptosporidiosis outbreak occurred in Milwaukee, Wisconsin, USA. An estimated 403,000 people became ill, including 4,400 people hospitalised. An estimated 69 people died during the outbreak, according to the CDC.

The UK's biggest outbreak occurred in Torbay in Devon in 1995.

In the summer of 1996, *Cryptosporidium* affected approximately 2,000 people in Cranbrook, British Columbia, Canada. Weeks later, a separate incident occurred in Kelowna, British Columbia, where 10,000 to 15,000 people got sick. In April 2001, an outbreak occurred in the city of North Battleford, Saskatchewan, Canada. Between 5800 and 7100 people suffered from diarrheal illness, and 1907 cases of cryptosporidiosis were confirmed. Equipment failures at the city's antiquated water filtration plant following maintenance were found to have caused the outbreak.

In the summer of 2005, after numerous reports by patrons of gastrointestinal upset, a water park at Seneca Lake State Park, in the Finger Lakes region of upstate New York, USA was found to have two water storage tanks infected with *Cryptosporidium*. By early September 2005, over 3,800 people reported symptoms of a *Cryptosporidium* infection. The "Sprayground" was ordered closed for the season on 15 August.

In October 2005, the Gwynedd and Anglesey areas of North Wales (UK) suffered an outbreak of cryptosporidiosis. The outbreak may have been linked to the drinking water supply from Llyn Cwellyn, but this is not yet confirmed. As a result, 231 people fell ill and the company Welsh Water (Dwr Cymru) advised 61,000 people to boil their water before use.

In March 2007, a suspected outbreak occurred in Galway, Ireland, after the source of water for much of the county, Lough Corrib, was suspected to be contaminated with the parasite. A large population (90,000 people), including areas of both Galway City and County, were advised to boil water for drinking, food preparation and for brushing teeth. On 21 March 2007, it was confirmed that the city and county's water supply was contaminated with the parasite. The area's water supply was finally given approval on 20 August 2007, five months after *Cryptosporidium* was first detected. Around 240 people are known to have contracted the disease; experts say the true figure could be up to 5,000.

Hundreds of public pools in 20 Utah, USA counties were closed to young children in 2007, as children under 5 are most likely to spread the disease, especially children wearing diapers. As of 10 September 2007 the Utah Department of Health had reported 1302 cases of cryptosporidiosis in the year; a more usual number would be 30. On 25 September the pools were reopened to those not requiring diapers, but hyperchlorination requirements were not lifted.

On 21 September 2007, a *Cryptosporidium* outbreak attacked the Western United States: 230 Idaho residents, with hundreds across the Rocky Mountain area; in the Boise and Meridian areas; Utah, 1,600 illnesses; Colorado and other Western states - Montana, decrease.

On 25 June 2008, *Cryptosporidium* was found in England in water supplies in Northampton, Daventry and some surrounding areas supplied from the Pitsford Reservoir, as reported on the BBC. People in the affected areas were warned not to drink tap water unless it had been boiled. Anglian Water confirmed that 108,000 households were affected, about 250,000 people. They advised that water might not be fit for human consumption for many weeks. The boil notice was lifted for all the affected customers on 4 July 2008.

Throughout the summer of 2008; many public swimming areas, water parks, and public pools in the Dallas/Fort Worth Metroplex of Texas, USA suffered an outbreak of cryptosporidiosis. Burger's Lake in Fort Worth was the first to report such an outbreak. This prompted some, if not all, city-owned and private pools to close and hyperchlorinate. To date, there have been 400 reported cases of *Cryptosporidium*.

In September 2008, a gym in Cambridge, UK was forced to close its swimming pool until further notice after health inspectors found an outbreak of cryptosporidiosis. Environmental Health authorities requested that the water be tested after it was confirmed that a young man had been infected.

In May 2010, the Behana creek water supply south of Cairns, Australia, was found to be contaminated by cryptosporidium.

In July 2010, a local sport centre in Cumbernauld (Glasgow, UK) detected traces of cryptosporidium in its swimming pools, causing a temporarily closure of the swimming pools.

In November 2010, over 4000 cases of cryptosporidiosis were reported in Östersund, Sweden. The source of contamination was the tap water. In mid December 2010 the number of reported cases was 12,400 according to local media.

As of April 2011, there has been an ongoing outbreak in Skellefteå, Sweden. Although many people have been diagnosed with cryptosporidiosis, the source of the parasite has not yet been found. Several tests have been taken around the water treatment unit "Abborren", but so far no results have turned up positive. Residents are being advised to boil the tap water as they continue to search for the contaminating source.

Since May 2011, there has been an ongoing outbreak in South Roscommon in Ireland. Although many people have been diagnosed with cryptosporidiosis, the source of the parasite has not yet been found. Testing continues and Roscommon County Council are now considering introducing Ultra Violet Filtration to their water treatment process in the next 12 months. Residents are being advised to boil the tap water and there is no sign of this boil notice being lifted in the near future.

Zoalene

Zoalene (dinitolmide) is a fodder additive for poultry, used to prevent coccidiosis infections. It is also known under trade names such as Coccidine A, Coccidot, and Zoamix.

Zoalene is usually added to feed in doses of 125 ppm (preventive) or 250 ppm (curative). It is a broad-spectrum anticoccidial drug, preventing seven main strains of *Eimeria coccidium*. It leaves no residues in tissues. It can be also used to prevent coccidiosis of domestic rabbits.

If zoalene is held at 120-125 °C for 24 hours or longer, it may react and self-heat and even explode.

Chapter 4

Strategies for Protecting Poultry from Coccidia

If ever organisms lived up to the label "parasite," it is those belonging to the order Coccidia.

Not only do the single-cell protozoans of the *Eimeria* genus infest the nation's poultry flocks, costing American producers an estimated $600 million-plus annually in medication costs and lost production; they also invade and take shelter in the very cells marshaled by the chicken's immune system to defeat them.

Though a vaccine is available in this country against coccidiosis, its key ingredient is a low dose of the live parasite, which stimulates protective immunity. But Hyun S. Lillehoj, who is an immunologist with the ARS Immunology and Disease Resistance Laboratory at Beltsville, Maryland, says the presence of the live parasite may pose problems.

"The live parasite can cause disease in the bird," Lillehoj contends. "If the bird's immune system isn't functioning properly for some reason, the live parasite in the vaccine can overcome the immune system. Also, there can be a negative interaction within the bird with feed contaminants such as mycotoxins or with other infections that might be present, such as *salmonella* or *campylobacter*."

Complicating the vaccine situation is the existence of seven different species of *Eimeria*.

"An effective vaccine needs to incorporate elements from all seven species," says Lillehoj. "The vaccine that has the live parasite uses many of the seven strains. But the incidence of variant species of *Eimeria* in the field is increasing, and the live coccidia vaccine cannot protect effectively against all of them. It's also very labour-intensive to produce the live parasites."

Lillehoj favours a different approach. She and her research team including support scientist Marjorie B. Nichols and technician Melody B. Lowe have devised a two-pronged strategy to thwart coccidia.

"The chicken's immune system produces cytotoxic T-cells whose function it is to target and destroy infected cells," explains Lillehoj. "That's part of nature's protective immune mechanism against this parasite.

"But there is a phase of the coccidia life cycle when the parasites are called sporozoites. These actually get inside the cytotoxic cells, which then cannot kill them, but instead deliver the parasites to the part of the intestine called the crypt epithelium, where they exit to develop."

Once nestled in crypt epithelial cells, the thriving coccidia wreak havoc in the intestinal lining and interfere with the chicken's ability to absorb nutrients from the feed it has eaten. Result: The bird doesn't gain weight and may die.

In 1993, Lillehoj and ARS immunologist James M. Trout observed coccidia's commandeering of cytotoxic cells firsthand when they used two fluorescent, colour-stained monoclonal antibodies to cling to and track movement of both parasites and cytotoxic cells inside chicken intestines.

Green-stained monoclonal antibodies allowed them to see where the coccidia went; red-stained antibodies pinpointed the presence of the cytotoxic cells. Overlapping red and green colours proved the coccidia invaded the very cells that were supposed to protect the chicken against them.

Part of Lillehoj's plan is to block the initial invasion of those crucial infection-fighting cytotoxic cells by the coccidia.

"The sporozoite has to bind to the cytotoxic cell to get inside it," she explains. "Once it binds, it makes a little dent on the cell. The parasite has a retractable structure called a conoid that makes this dent. Then enzymes from the parasite act on the cell to make an opening for the parasite to get in.

"We've developed and have applied for a patent on a chicken monoclonal antibody that identifies a protein that the sporozoite uses to cling to the cytotoxic cell. In laboratory tests, this antibody actually blocks the sporozoite invasion of the cytotoxic cell."

Lillehoj is working with ARS molecular biologists Mark C. Jenkins and Kang D. Choi on ways to use the protein recognised by the antibody as a potential vaccine. Also promising as potential weapons are cytokines, substances produced naturally by the bird's white blood cells.

We have shown in laboratory tests that some cytokines inhibit development of the parasite," says Lillehoj.

"They also enhance cytotoxic activity by turning precursor cytotoxic cells into active cytotoxic cells. Once activated, these cytotoxic cells kill parasite-infected host cells. Cytokines also activate white blood cells called macrophages to devour the parasites."

Starting in 1995, Lillehoj collaborated with ARS molecular biologist Dante S. Zarlenga and scientists at Korea's Seoul National University to clone the chicken gene that controls manufacture of a cytokine called gamma-interferon. The research team has produced genetically engineered chicken gamma-interferon and is testing its protective powers in live chickens. Early results look promising, Lillehoj says.

"If this works, a bird that's treated with the gamma-interferon might still get infected with coccidia, but it might not lose as much weight or get as bad a case of coccidiosis," she explains. "You wouldn't want to completely block the infection, anyway, because then you wouldn't stimulate the bird's immune system to provide natural immunity against future coccidia infections or other opportunistic pathogens."

Gamma-interferon may prove useful in the battle against coccidia in other ways as well, Lillehoj adds.

"Antigens are proteins from the parasite that stimulate an immune response from an animal's immune system," she points out. "It's been shown in mammalian cells that when you add gamma-interferon to a weak antigen, you get a greater immune response than if you just vaccinate with the antigen alone. Plans are under way to use gamma-interferon as an adjuvant to enhance the action of the vaccine."

Mass production of gamma-interferon may be tricky, Lillehoj says. In lab tests, attempts to reproduce the substance by inserting the gene for its production into fast-multiplying *E. coli* bacteria fell short of the scientists' expectations.

"The protein was not very effective when expressed in *E. coli*," Lillehoj admits. "But once you have a gene that expresses the protein, you can raise it in a mammalian cell line." One possible solution to the protection dilemma might be to identify an antigen common to all strains of coccidia and use that as the basis for a new vaccine.

"We know of one such segment, but we're not ready to test it yet as a vaccine," says Lillehoj.

The more common game plan—waiting to clean up coccidiosis in flocks after it occurs—is rapidly becoming a risky proposition, according to Lillehoj.

"The major problem is that the parasite develops drug resistance very quickly," she notes. "The main emphasis for control has been on drugs, but the coccidia have developed resistance to all the drugs ever tested against them."

The ARS research team's multifaceted efforts come down to one simple goal: to mimic nature.

"In the field, once birds have been exposed to coccidia, they develop immunity," says Lillehoj. "We've been trying to figure out how chickens get that immunity. Over the years, we've learned a lot about how the parasite invades cells and stimulates natural immunity." — By Sandy Miller Hays, ARS.

Hyun S. Lillehoj is at the USDA ARS Immunology and Disease Resistance Laboratory, Bldg. 1043, 10300 Baltimore Ave., Beltsville, MD 20705-2350; phone (301) 504-6170.

"Two Strategies for Protecting Poultry From Coccidia" was published in the October 1996 issue of *Agricultural Research* magazine.

Common Cold

The common cold (also known as nasopharyngitis, acute viral rhinopharyngitis, acute coryza, or a cold) (Latin: *rhinitis acuta catarrhalis*) is a viral infectious disease of the upper respiratory system, caused primarily by rhinoviruses and coronaviruses. Common symptoms include a cough, sore throat, runny nose, and fever. There is no cure for the common cold, but symptoms usually resolve in 7 to 10 days, with some symptoms possibly lasting for up to three weeks.

The common cold is the most frequent infectious disease in humans with the average adult contracting two to four infections a year and the average child contracting between 6 and 12. Collectively, colds, influenza, and other upper respiratory tract infections (URTI) with similar symptoms are included in the diagnosis of influenza-like illness.

Signs and Symptoms

Symptoms are cough, sore throat, runny nose, and nasal congestion; sometimes this may be accompanied by conjunctivitis (pink eye), muscle aches, fatigue, headaches, shivering, and loss of appetite.

Fever is often present thus creating a symptom picture which overlaps with influenza. The symptoms of influenza however are usually more severe.

Those suffering from colds often report a sensation of chilliness even though the cold is not generally accompanied by fever, and although chills are generally associated with fever, the sensation may not always be caused by actual fever. In one study, 60% of those suffering from a sore throat and upper respiratory tract infection reported headaches, often due to nasal congestion.

Progression

The viral replication begins 2 to 6 hours after initial contact. Symptoms usually begin 2 to 5 days after initial infection but occasionally occur in as little as 10 hours. Symptoms peak 2–3 days after symptom onset, whereas influenza symptom onset is constant and immediate. The symptoms usually resolve spontaneously in 7 to 10 days but some can last for up to three weeks. In children the cough lasts for more than 10 days in 35–40% of cases and continues for more than 25 days in 10%.

The first indication of an upper respiratory virus is often a sore or scratchy throat. Other common symptoms are runny nose, congestion, and sneezing. These are sometimes accompanied by muscle aches, fatigue, malaise, headache, weakness, or loss of appetite. Cough and fever generally indicate influenza rather than an upper respiratory virus with a positive predictive value of around 80%. Symptoms may be more severe in infants and young children, and in these cases it may include fever and hives. Upper respiratory viruses may also be more severe in smokers.

Infectious Period

Researchers have studied rhinovirus-caused colds more than other colds. Rhinovirus-caused colds are most infectious during the first three days of symptoms. They become much less infectious after those three days.

Cause

Viruses

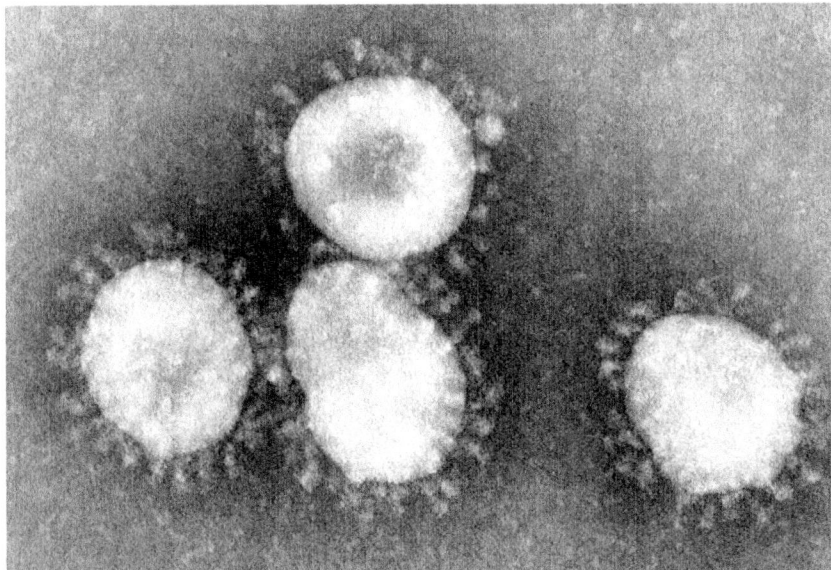

Figure : Coronaviruses are a group of viruses known for causing the common cold. They have a halo, or crown-like (corona) appearance when viewed under an electron microscope.

The common cold is a viral infection of the upper respiratory tract. The most commonly implicated virus is a rhinovirus (30–50%), a type of picornavirus with 99 known serotypes. Others include: coronavirus (10–15%), influenza (5–15%), human parainfluenza viruses, human respiratory syncytial virus, adenoviruses, enteroviruses, and metapneumovirus.

In total over 200 serologically different viral types cause colds. Coronaviruses are particularly implicated in adult colds. Of over 30 coronaviruses, 3 or 4 cause infections in humans, but they are difficult to grow in the laboratory and their significance is thus less well-understood. Due to the many different types of viruses and their tendency for continuous mutation, it is impossible to gain complete immunity to the common cold.

Risk Factors

Touching eyes, nose, or mouth with contaminated fingers. This behaviour increases the likelihood of transferring viruses from the surface of the hands, where they are harmless, into the upper respiratory tract, where they can infect the tissues. It has been demonstrated that cold viruses can be spread by touching contaminated objects and surfaces, or by brief contact of hands.

Spending time in an enclosed area with an infected person or in close contact with an infected person. Common colds are droplet-borne infections, which means that they can be transmitted through breathing in tiny particles that the infected person emits when he or she coughs or sneezes. In one study, the virus was recovered in 1/13 of sneezes and 0/8 coughs generated by adults with natural rhinovirus (cold) infections.

The role of body cooling in causing the common cold is controversial. It is the most commonly offered folk explanation for the disease, and it has received some experimental evidence. One study showed that exposure to the cold causes cold symptoms in about 10% of those exposed, and that the subjects experiencing this effect report far more colds overall than those who do not. However, a variety of other studies do not show such an effect.

A history of smoking extends the duration of illness by about three days.

Getting fewer than seven hours of sleep per night has been associated with a risk three times higher of developing an infection when exposed to a rhinovirus, compared to those who sleep more than eight hours per night.

Common colds are seasonal, occurring more frequently during winter outside of tropical zones. Some argue that this is partly due to a change in behaviours such as increased time spent indoors, which puts infected people in close proximity to other people, rather than the exposure to cold temperatures.

Low humidity increases viral transmission rates. One theory is that dry air causes evaporation of water, thus allowing small viral droplets to disperse farther and stay in the air longer.

Counterintuitively, people with stronger immune systems are more likely to develop symptomatic colds. This is because the symptoms of a cold are directly due to the strong immune response to the virus, not the virus itself. People with less active immune systems—about a quarter of adults—get infected with the viruses, but the relatively weak immunological response produces no significant or identifiable symptoms. These people are asymptomatic carriers and can unknowingly spread the virus to other people. Because strong immune responses cause cold symptoms, "boosting" the immune system increases cold symptoms.

Pathophysiology

The common cold is a type of pharyngitis (inflammation of the throat). In the common cold, the inflammation is caused by a viral infection in the uppermost part of the throat (the nasopharynx), which runs from behind the nose down to the mouth.

The common cold virus is transmitted mainly from contact with saliva or nasal secretions of an infected person, either directly, when a healthy person breathes in the virus-laden aerosol generated when an infected person coughs or sneezes, or by touching a contaminated surface and then touching the nose or eyes.

Symptoms are not necessary for viral shedding or transmission, as a percentage of asymptomatic subjects exhibit viruses in nasal swabs. It is generally not possible to identify the virus type through symptoms, although influenza can be distinguished by its sudden onset, fever, and cough.

The major entry point for the virus is normally the nose, but can also be the eyes (in this case drainage into the nasopharynx would occur through the nasolacrimal duct). From there, it is transported to the back of the nose and the adenoid area. The virus then attaches to a receptor, ICAM-1, which is located on the surface of cells of the lining of the nasopharynx. The receptor fits into a docking port on the surface of the virus. Large amounts of virus receptor are present on cells of the adenoid. After attachment to the receptor, virus is taken into the cell, where it starts an infection, and increases ICAM-1 production, which in turn helps the immune response against the virus. Rhinovirus colds do not generally cause damage to the nasal epithelium. Macrophages trigger the production of cytokines, which in combination with mediators cause the symptoms. Cytokines cause the systemic effects. The mediator bradykinin plays a major role in causing the local symptoms such as sore throat and nasal irritation.

The common cold is self-limiting, and the host's immune system effectively deals with the infection. Within a few days, the body's humoral immune response begins producing specific antibodies that can prevent the virus from infecting cells. Additionally, as part of the cell-mediated immune response, leukocytes destroy the virus through phagocytosis and destroy infected cells to prevent further viral replication. In healthy, immunocompetent individuals, the common cold resolves in seven days on average.

Prevention

The best prevention for the common cold is staying away from people who are infected, and places where infected individuals have been.

Regular hand washing is recommended to reduce transmission of cold viruses and other pathogens via direct contact. Virus can be recovered from the hands of <"40% of adults with rhinovirus colds, and the quantity of virus recovered from the hands is also generally greater than that recovered in coughs and sneezes. Washing of the hands reduces virus count on the skin.

Hand washing with plain soap and water is recommended. The mechanical action of hand rubbing with plain soap, rinsing, and drying physically removes the virus particles from the hands.

Alcohol-based hand sanitizers provide very little protection against upper respiratory infections, especially among children.

Because the common cold is caused by a virus instead of a bacterium, antibacterial soaps are no better than regular soap for removing the virus from skin or other surfaces.

Aqueous iodine has been found to reliably eliminate the cold virus on human skin, however iodine is not acceptable for general use as a virucidal hand treatment because it discolours and dries the skin.

Randomised controlled trials have shown that hand washing using different combinations of cleaning agents resulted in a reduction in the incidence of rhinovirus infections. In two studies at day care facilities, increased handwashing of caregivers reduced the incidence of colds in children by up to 20%. However, scheduled handwashing at an elementary school has been shown to reduce the incidence of all communicable illnesses and gastrointestinal illnesses in particular, but was not shown to prevent respiratory ailments.

Efforts to develop a vaccine against the common cold have been unsuccessful. Common colds are produced by a large variety of rapidly mutating viruses; successful creation of a broadly effective vaccine is highly improbable. Exposure to cold temperatures and dry weather have been found to facilitate viral infection, explaining why colds and flu are more prevalent in winter outside of tropical areas. Cold weather may make the mucous lining of the respiratory tract more sluggish, taking longer to sweep any inhaled virus particles away. This allows more time for the virus to establish infection and means an individual is infectious (exhaling virus particles) for longer. In humidity above 80%, droplets containing viruses fall out of the air.

However, whilst it creates a better environment for the virus, cold weather itself does not directly cause colds and neither is there evidence supporting the idea that cold weather weakens the cells involved in the immune response.

Management

There are currently no medications or herbal remedies which have been conclusively demonstrated to shorten the duration of infection in all people with cold symptoms.

Treatment comprises symptomatic support usually via analgesics for fever, headache, sore muscles, and sore throat.

Symptomatic

Treatments that help alleviate symptoms include simple analgesics and antipyretics such as ibuprofen and acetaminophen/paracetamol. Evidence does not show that cough medicine is any more effective than simple analgesics and is not recommended for use in children due to a lack of evidence supporting its effectiveness and the potential for harm.

Symptoms of a runny nose can be reduced by a first generation antihistamine; however, it can cause drowsiness and other side effects. Other decongestants such as pseudoephedrine are effective in adults but there is insufficient evidence to support their use in children. Anticholinergics such as Ipratropium nasal spray can reduce the symptoms of runny nose with less side effects.

One study has found chest vapour rub to be effective at providing some symptomatic relief of nocturnal cough, congestion, and sleep difficulty.

Getting plenty of rest, drinking fluids to maintain hydration, and gargling with warm salt water, are reasonable conservative measures. Evidence for encouraging the active intake of fluids in acute respiratory infections is lacking as is the use of heated humidified air. Saline nasal drops may help alleviate nasal congestion.

Antibiotics and Antivirals

Antibiotics have no effect against viral infections and thus have no effect against the viruses that cause the common cold and due to their side effects cause overall harm. There are no approved antiviral drugs for the common cold even though some preliminary research has shown benefit.

Alternative Treatments

While many alternative treatments are used there is insufficient scientific evidence to support the use of most. Honey may be effective treatment in decreasing cough and improving sleep in children more than no treatment or dextromethorphan. However, honey should not be given to a child younger than one year old because of the risk of infant botulism. The benefits versus risk of nasal irrigation are currently unclear and therefore it is not recommended.

Zinc deficiency impairs immune function. It has been suggested that zinc may inhibit rhinovirus replication and reduce inflammation. Trials have found that zinc supplements can somewhat reduce the severity and duration of common cold symptoms when taken by otherwise healthy adults within 24 hours of onset of symptoms.

Vitamin C's effect on the common cold has been extensively researched. It has not been shown effective in prevention or treatment of the common cold, except in limited circumstances (specifically, individuals exercising vigorously in cold environments). Routine vitamin C supplementation does not reduce the incidence or severity of the common cold in the general population, though it may reduce the duration of illness.

Evidence about the usefulness of echinacea supplements, a popular herbal remedy, is contradictory. Well-conducted research studies tend to have negative results at a much higher rate than poorly conducted studies. Different types of echinacea supplements may vary in their effectiveness.

Generally, those studies that show supportive results indicate that echinacea might reduce the likelihood of developing cold symptoms upon inoculation with a virus by about half.

Prognosis

The common cold is generally mild and self-limiting.

Pneumonia is a possible complication.

Epidemiology

Upper respiratory tract infections are the most common infectious diseases among adults, who have two to four respiratory infections annually. Children may have six to ten colds a year (and up to 12 colds a year for school children). In the United States, the incidence of colds is higher in the fall (autumn) and winter, with most infections occurring between September and April. The seasonality may be due to the start of the school year, or due to people spending more time indoors (thus in closer proximity with each other) increasing the chance of transmission of the virus.

History

The name "common cold" came into use in the 16th century, due to the similarity between its symptoms and those of exposure to cold weather. Norman Moore relates in his history of the Study of Medicine that James I continually suffered from nasal colds, which were then thought to be caused by polypi, sinus trouble, or autotoxaemia.

In the 18th century, Benjamin Franklin considered the causes and prevention of the common cold. After several years of research he concluded: "People often catch cold from one another when shut up together in small close rooms, coaches, etc. and when sitting near and conversing so as to breathe in each other's transpiration."

Although viruses had not yet been discovered, Franklin hypothesized that the common cold was passed between people through the air. He recommended exercise, bathing, and moderation in food and drink consumption to avoid the common cold. Franklin's theory on the transmission of the cold was confirmed some 150 years later.

Common Cold Unit

In the United Kingdom, the Common Cold Unit was set up by the Medical Research Council in 1946. The unit worked with volunteers who were infected with various viruses. The rhinovirus was discovered there. In the late 1950s, researchers were able to grow one of these cold viruses in a tissue culture, as it would not grow in fertilised chicken eggs, the method used for many other viruses. In the 1970s, the CCU demonstrated that treatment with interferon during the incubation phase of rhinovirus infection protects somewhat against the disease, but no practical treatment could be developed. The unit was closed in 1989, two years after it completed research of zinc gluconate lozenges in the prophylaxis and treatment of rhinovirus colds, the only successful treatment in the history of the unit.

Social and Cultural

Economics

In the United States, the common cold leads to 75 to 100 million physician visits annually at a conservative cost estimate of $7.7 billion per year. Americans spend $2.9 billion on over-the-counter drugs and another $400 million on prescription medicines for symptomatic relief.

More than one-third of patients who saw a doctor received an antibiotic prescription, which has implications for antibiotic resistance from overuse of such drugs.

An estimated 22 to 189 million school days are missed annually due to a cold. As a result, parents missed 126 million workdays to stay home to care for their children. When added to the 150 million workdays missed by employees suffering from a cold, the total economic impact of cold-related work loss exceeds $20 billion per year. This accounts for 40% of time lost from work.

Legal

Canada in 2009 restricted the use of over-the-counter cough and cold medication in children 6 years and under due to concerns regarding risks and unproven benefits.

Cold Weather

The traditional folk theory is that a cold can be "caught" by prolonged exposure to cold weather such as rain or winter conditions, which is where the disease got its name. Common colds are seasonal in temperate latitudes, with more occurring during winter. The experimental evidence for this effect is uneven: many experiments have failed to produce evidence that short-term exposure to cold weather or direct chilling increases susceptibility to infection, implying that the seasonal variation is instead due to a change in behaviours such as increased time spent indoors at close proximity to others. However, other experiments do find such an effect for both body chilling and cold air exposure, and a number of mechanisms by which lower temperatures could compromise the immune system have been suggested, while other experiments have shown that exposure to cold temperatures may instead stimulate the immune system.

Research

Dermanyssus Gallinae

Dermanyssus gallinae (also known as the red mite, poultry mite, red poultry mite and chicken mite) is an ectoparasite of poultry and other bird species.

Description

The mites are blood feeders and attack resting birds at night. They are generally white or greyish in colour, becoming darker or redder when engorged with blood. After feeding, they hide in cracks and crevices away from daylight, where they mate and lay eggs. The mite progresses through 5 life stages: egg, larva, protonymph, deutonymph and adult. Under favourable conditions this life cycle can be completed within seven days, so populations can grow rapidly - causing anaemia in badly affected flocks of poultry.

Young birds are most susceptible. The mites can also affect the health of the birds indirectly, as they may serve as vectors for diseases such as Salmonellosis, avian spirochaetosis and *Erysipelothrix rhusiopathiae*.

Dermansyssus gallinae can also feed on some species of mammals, including humans, - causing dermatitis and skin lesions. However the mite needs an avian host to reproduce.

Clinical Signs and Diagnosis

The mites normally feed around the breast and legs of hens, causing pain, irritation, and a decrease in egg production. Pustules, scabs, hyperpigmentation and feather loss may develop.

If they are present in large numbers, *D. gallinae* can cause anaemia in hens which presents as pallor of the comb and wattle.

A presumptive diagnosis can be made in flocks of laying hens, usually based on a history of decreasing egg production, anaemia and mortalities in young or ill birds. Definitive diagnosis is only achieved following identification of eggs, faeces or the mites themselves

Treatment and Prevention

Ectoparasiticides can be used to treat affected poultry. These chemical controls, if used, should be used in rotation to avoid the build up of resistance. Red mites can survive for up to 10 months in an empty hen house. Creosote treatment of wood will kill mites.

The Poultry Red Mite, Dermanyssus Gallinae, A Potential Vector of Erysipelothrix Rhusiopathiae Causing Erysipelas in Hens

Egg Binding

In farming, aviculture and animal husbandry, the term egg binding refers to a medical condition in birds where the female is unable to pass an egg that has formed. The egg may be stuck near the cloaca, or further inside. Egg binding is a reasonably common, and potentially serious, condition that can lead to infection or damage to internal tissue. The bound egg may be gently massaged out; failing this it may become necessary to break the egg *in situ* and remove it in parts. If broken, the oviduct should be cleaned of shell fragments and egg residue to avoid damage or infection.

The term can also be seen in herpetoculture, as this condition can occur in female reptiles. It is inadvisable to attempt to break a reptile egg to remove it from an egg bound female. This procedure may be done by a veterinarian, who will insert a needle into the egg, and withdraw the contents with a syringe, allowing the egg to collapse and be removed. Nonsurgical interventions include administering oxytocin to improve contractions and allow the eggs to pass normally. In many cases, egg bound reptiles must undergo surgery to have stuck eggs removed.

Egg binding in reptiles is quickly fatal if left untreated, therefore gravid females who become very lethargic and cease feeding, need immediate medical treatment in order to treat the potentially life-threatening condition. A recent episode of the Animal Planet reality show E-Vet Interns featured the treatment of an egg bound turtle named Napoleon. Exotics specialist Dr. Kevin Fitzgerald of Alameda East Veterinary Hospital is shown treating her with oxytocin and then eventually having to resort to surgery with footage of the large number of eggs that were removed. Dr. Fitzgerald was shown explaining to the new interns how dangerous this condition can be for a pet turtle and the need for early medical intervention.

Egg binding can occur if an egg is malformed and/or too large, the animal is weakened by illness, improper husbandry, or stress, or if hormonal balances are wrong (producing weak contractions). Factors that can contribute to the risk of egg binding include calcium deficiency, breeding animals that are too young or too small, not providing suitable laying areas (leading to deliberate retention of eggs), and overfeeding of species in which clutch size is dependent on food intake (such as Veiled Chameleons).

Egg Binding

You first generally notice this ailment rather too late, when it is obvious the hen is in some discomfort. The hen often stands or moves in an odd way, usually with her tail held very low and her rear end tucked between her legs. Sometimes they just sit around looking ruffled, but often it is obvious the bird is straining to pass an egg. If you spot it early your chances of helping the hen are greatest.

Egg binding can happen in young hens just starting to lay or in older birds that have become fat. Lack of exercise can cause fat to build up in the birds body, around the reproductive organs and so cause the egg to get stuck. Lack of calcium in the diet can be a major cause of it. Sometimes the egg is just too large for the bird to pass, sometimes the shell is rough and not easily expelled.

In my experience the egg bound hen, (Unless it's a pullet first starting to lay, these seem to respond better) has not got a very good outlook. If you approach the problem with this in mind then anything you can do to save your bird is a bonus. Unless the egg gets passed without too much fuss, it frequently seems to cause the bird massive shock, the bird often will die. Egg binding can also cause a prolapse, which will forever cause problems with that hen afterwards. However going on the principle that if its going to die without help. You have to try something!

So here are some things you can do to assist the hen, and are always worth trying, especially on a young bird who is just having trouble with her first egg. These birds are usually the most rewarding to treat, they seem to respond better and often it does not reoccur with them, unlike older birds who have developed internal problems.

The first thing to do is to put the bird somewhere warm for a while, often, this treatment in itself can help enormously. As with many bird related ailments, heat can be a wonderful healer. If the hen is in shock from it is vital. A comfortable heat will often give the bird enough of a boost to be able to pass the egg herself. Hopefully this will be the case with your bird. If after a while she is still straining and no egg has arrived, I would suggest gently introducing some slightly warmed oil (body temp) into the vent, cooking oil is fine. If the egg is visible hold the hen vent downwards over a bowl of gently steaming water.. (Don't over-heat the poor thing she's going through hell as it is!)

Many people will tell you that if you break the egg the hen will die. Yes this is very often the case, sometimes the act of breaking the egg may cause the bird to just have a heart attack and drop dead. I've seen it happen, but I have had success on two occasions using this method. I gently and carefully made a small hole in the visible end of the egg, and emptied the contents. The contractions of the hen quickly crushed the now empty shell and I pulled it free. DO NOT leave any egg behind!

If your hen finally lays her egg she will show immediate and understandable relief! I always give the hen some electrolytes to drink and a light feed and usually they are happy to go back to the flock after a brief rest. In the case of an older bird, I usually put her on a light diet for a few days to try to bring her out of lay. Especially if I think it is due to the hen being overweight.

Now for some modern stuff that I have heard about but haven't tried, but I'm absolutely going to ask my vet about! I have recently heard that excellent results can be obtained very quickly with injectable calcium gluconate which is given as an inter muscular injection into the pectoral muscle. I want to find out more about this as it could be very useful in future.

Preventing Egg Binding

I have found that by using a calcium/mineral supplement added to the birds layers rations a couple of times a week that this problem has decreased. I have a lot of birds and generally used to expect to have a couple of cases of egg binding during the season. The last couple of years its been very minor, if at all, so I think that the added calcium/minerals may have just given that extra help needed to help prevent this ailment. As calcium is required for the muscle contractions which push the egg out of the body as well as for the formation of the shell I think extra calcium and minerals are a very good idea during the breeding season. I for one will not rely on breeders pellets and oyster shell alone.

Fatty Liver Hemorrhagic Syndrome

Fatty liver hemorrhagic syndrome (also referred to as fatty liver syndrome), a disease in chickens and other birds, affects only hens (females). Birds with this disease have large amounts of fat deposited in their liver and abdomen.

This often results in an enlarged liver that is easily damaged and prone to bleeding. In some cases the disease is fatal, usually as a result of blood loss from an internal hemorrhage in the liver. The hemorrhage often occurs when a hen is straining to lay her egg. Fatty liver hemorrhagic syndrome is "the major cause of mortality in laying hens."

Causes

Excessive dietary energy intake is believed to be the cause of fatty liver hemorrhagic syndrome. Heredity may also play a role, but it is not the entire cause for the disease. Birds housed in cages will more likely be affected because they are unable to exercise to burn off the extra dietary energy.

Walking hens are less likely to develop this problem. The disease is observed most often in birds that appear to be healthy and in a state of high egg production. As a result, death can occur quite unexpectedly.

Symptoms

Affected birds are usually overweight and may also have pale combs. Generally, however, the disease has few or no symptoms prior to the bird's death.

Treatment

The use of L-Tryptophan in the diet can decrease the syndrome.

Fowlpox

Fowlpox is a worldwide disease of poultry caused by viruses of the family *Poxviridae* and the genus *Avipoxvirus*. The viruses causing fowlpox are distinct from one another but antigenically similar, possible hosts including chickens, turkeys, quail, canaries, pigeons, and many other species of birds.

There are two forms of the disease. The first is spread by biting insects (especially mosquitoes) and wound contamination and causes lesions on the comb, wattles, and beak. Birds affected by this form usually recover within a few weeks. The second form is spread by inhalation of the virus and causes a diphtheritic membrane to form in the mouth, pharynx, larynx, and sometimes the trachea. The prognosis for this form is poor.

Vaccines are available for fowlpox (ATCvet code: QI01AD12). Chicken are usually vaccinated with *pigeonpox virus*. Turkeys are also routinely vaccinated.

Turkeypox

Turkeypox is a virus of the family *Poxviridae* and the genus *Avipoxvirus*. It is one of the most common diseases in the Wild Turkey (Meleagris gallopavo) population.

Causes

Turkeypox is caused by the fowlpox virus, which infects birds.

Turkeypox, like all avipoxviruses, is transmitted either through skin contact or by arthropods (typically mosquitos) acting as mechanical vectors.

Gallid Herpesvirus 1

Gallid herpesvirus 1 (GaHV-1) (also known as Avian herpesvirus 1) is a virus of the family *Herpesviridae* that causes avian infectious laryngotracheitis. It was originally recognised as a disease of chickens in the United States in 1926. The disease also occurs in pheasants.

The disease is usually referred to as Infectious laryngotracheitis or simply LT in the poultry industry.

It is widely viewed as one of the most contagious viruses that affect the poultry industry. A confirmed case will usually result in the establishment of a quarantine zone around the farm. Inside this quarantine zone, poultry workers will avoid poultry farms to prevent the spread of the virus.

GaHV-1 is shed in respiratory secretions and transmitted by droplet inhalation or via fomites. A previously unexposed flock will develop cases for two to eight weeks following introduction. The incubation period is two to eight days.

Clinical Signs and Diagnosis

Symptoms include coughing, sneezing, head shaking, lethargy, discharge from the eyes and nostrils (sometimes bloody), and difficulty breathing. The name comes from the severe inflammation of the larynx and trachea. A diphtheritic membrane may form in the trachea, causing obstruction.

There may be problems in egg laying and the production of abnormal or thin-shelled eggs.

Mortality is typically less than 15 percent.

Histopathology, PCR, ELISA, immunofluorescent staining and viral isolation are all possible methods of diagnosis.

Treatment and Control

A vaccine is available (ATCvet code: QI01AD08), but it does not prevent latent infections. It can be used during an outbreak to decrease morbidity and deaths.

Biosecurity measure including quarantine, isolation and disinfection are very important in controlling the spread of an outbreak.

Chapter 5

Avian Infectious Laryngotracheitis

Introduction

Gallid Herpes virus causes respiratory disease in chickens and pheasants.

Disease varies from mild to peracute, with mortality in peracute outbreaks exceeding 50%. As with all herpesviruses, GHV-1 can remain latent in carriers after infection and then be shed intermittently, recrudescing with stress.

Signalment

The chicken is the primary host and reservoir host. A form of LT has been described in pheasants.

Distribution

Worldwide. Transmission is via direct contact and contaminated people and equipment. Vermin and wild birds and dogs may aid mechanical transmission.

Clinical Signs

Respiratory signs:

- Nasal discharge which is often bloody
- Coughing which may also include blood
- Sneezing, dyspnoea, gasping, upper respiratory tract pain
- Abnormal lung sounds
- Decreased egg production, thin egg shells, lack of growth
- Neurological and ophthalmologic signs may develop.

Death may occur rapidly and with high mortality in peracute and acute disease. In recent times, LT usually presents in a mild form and most birds recover.

Diagnosis

On post-mortem, haemorrhagic tracheitis and bloodstained mucus are evident. Pneumonia and sacculitis may also be seen. Caseous diptheritic membranes may be present on the mucosae of the upper respiratory tract.

Histopathology reveals loss of cilia, mucosal gland atrophy, intranuclear inclusion bodies and epithelial cell sloughing. Characteristic syncytia develop. A fibrinonecrotic membrane may be present in more chronic disease cases.

Antigen ELISA is both straightforward, quick and sensitive. The PCR can be used to detect LTV.

Immunofluorescent or Immunoperoxidase staining can also be performed and is more rapid but less sensitive.

Virus isolation on a variety of tissues including tracheal swabs or tissue samples may be useful.

Agar Gel Immunodiffusion can detect virus in tracheal samples.

Electron microscopy can be used to demonstrate viral particles in tracheal scrapings or exudates but is insensitive.

Measuring viral antibody measures infection indirectly as serum antibodies peak around 2 weeks after infection and wane slowly afterwards.

Treatment

Where early diagnosis is made, vaccination can be administered in the face of infection to help reduce further morbidity and mortality.

Control

ILT can be effectively controlled by vaccination. Vaccinated and unvaccinated birds should not be mixed due to the possibility of reversion to virulence. Most are modified live isolates and are administered by eye drop.

Adequate Biosecurity, Quarantine and Disinfection is also Essential. Wild birds and vermin should be prevented from accessing poultry and their food/water sources.

Gapeworm

A gapeworm (*Syngamus trachea*) is a parasitic nematode worm infecting the tracheas of certain birds. The resulting disease, known as gape or the gapes, occurs when the worms clog and obstruct the airway. The worms are also known as red worms or forked worms due to their red colour and the permanent procreative conjunction of males and females. Gapeworm is common in young, domesticated chickens and turkeys.

When the female gapeworm lays her eggs in the trachea of an infected bird, the eggs are coughed up, swallowed, then defecated. When birds consume the eggs found in the feces or an intermediate host such as earthworms, snails (*Planorbarius corneus, Bithynia tentaculata*, ...), or slugs, they become infected with the parasite.

Ivermectin is a drug often used to control gapeworm infection in birds.

Morphology

Males and females are joined together in a state of permanent copulation forming a Y shape "forked worm". They are also known as the "red worm" because of their colour. Females are much larger (up to 20 mm long) than males (up to 6 mm long). The life history of the gapeworm is peculiar in that transmission from bird to bird may be successfully accomplished either directly (by the feeding of embryonated eggs or infective larvae) or indirectly (by ingestion of earthworms containing free or encysted gapeworm larvae they had obtained by feeding on contaminated soil).

Life Cycle and Pathogenesis

The life cycle is complicated in both its preparasitic and parasitic phases. In the preparasitic phase, L3s develop inside the eggs at which time they may hatch. Earthworms play an important role in the life cycle, serving as transport (paratenic) hosts. Larvae have been shown to remain viable for more than three years encapsulated in earthworm muscles. Other invertebrates may also serve as paratenic hosts and these include terrestrial snails and slugs as well as the larvae of Musca domestica (the common house fly) and Lucilia sericata (the green bottle fly responsible for cutaneous myiasis). The parasitic phase involves substantial migration in the definitive host to reach the predilection site. Young birds are most severely affected with migration of larvae and adults through the lungs causing a severe pneumonia. Lymphoid nodules form at the point of attachment of the worms in the bronchi and trachea. Adult worms also appear to feed on blood. Worms in the bronchi and trachea provoke a hemorrhagic tracheitis and bronchitis with formation of large quantities of mucus, plugging the air passages and, in severe cases, causing asphyxiation. Pheasants appear to be particularly susceptible to infections resulting in mortality rates as high as 25% during outbreaks. The rapidly growing worms soon obstruct the lumen of the trachea and cause suffocation. Turkey poults, baby chicks and pheasant chicks are most susceptible to infection. Turkey poults usually develop gapeworm signs earlier and begin to die sooner after infection than young chickens. Lesions are usually found in the trachea of turkeys and pheasants but seldom if ever in the tracheas of young chickens and guinea fowl. The male worm, in the form of lesions, remains permanently attached to the tracheal wall throughout the duration of its life. The female worms apparently detach and reattach from time to time in order to obtain a more abundant supply of food.

Epidemiology

Earthworm transport hosts are important factors in the transmission of Syngamus trachea where poultry and game birds are reared on soil. The longevity of L3s in earthworms (up to 3 years) is particularly important in perpetuating the infection from year to year. Wild birds may serve as reservoirs of infection and have been implicated as the sources of infections in outbreaks on game-bird farms as well as poultry farms. Wild reservoir hosts may include pheasants, ruffed grouse, partridges, turkeys, magpies, meadowlarks, robins, grackles, jays, jackdaws, rooks, starlings and crows. There is also evidence to suggest that strains of Syngamus trachea from wild bird reservoir hosts may be more infective for domestic birds if they first pass through an earthworm transport host rather than by direct infections via ingestion of L3s or eggs containing L3s. Clinical signs Blockage of the bronchi and trachea with worms and mucus will cause infected birds to gasp for air. They stretch out their necks, open their mouths and gasp for air producing a hissing noise as they do so. This "gaping" posture has given rise to the common term "gapeworm" to describe Syngamus trachea. These clinical signs first appear approximately 1-2 weeks after infection. Birds infected with gapeworms show signs of weakness and emaciation and usually spend much of their time with eyes closed and head drawn back against the body. An infected bird may give its head a convulsive shake in an attempt to remove the obstruction from the trachea so that normal breathing may be resumed. Severely affected birds, particularly young ones, will deteriorate rapidly;

they stop drinking and become anorexic. At this stage, death is the usual outcome. Adult birds are usually less severely affected and may only show an occasional cough or even no obvious clinical signs.

Diagnosis

A diagnosis is usually made on the basis of the classical clinical signs of "gaping". Subclinical infections with few worms may be confirmed at necropsy by finding copulating worms in the trachea and also by finding the characteristic eggs in the feces of infected birds. Examination of the trachea of infection birds shows that the mucous membrane is extensively irritated and inflamed. Coughing is apparently the result of this irritation to the mucous lining.

Control and Treatment of Syngamus Trachea

Prevention

In the artificial rearing of pheasants, gapes are a serious menace. Confinement rearing of young birds has reduced the problem in chickens compared to a few years ago. However, this parasite continues to present an occasional problem with turkeys raised on range. Confinement rearing of broilers/pullets and caging of laying hens, have significantly influenced the quantity and variety of nematode infections in poultry. For most nematodes, control measures consist of sanitation and breaking the life cycle rather than chemotherapy. Confinement rearing on litter largely prevents infections with nematodes using intermediate hosts such as earthworms or grasshoppers, which are not normally found in poultry houses. Conversely, nematodes with direct life cycles or those that utilise intermediate hosts such as beetles, which are common in poultry houses, may prosper. Treatment of the soil or litter to kill intermediate hosts may be beneficial. Insecticides suitable for litter treatment include carbaryl, tetrachlorvinphos (stirofos). However, treatment is usually done only between grow-outs. Extreme care should be taken to ensure that feed and water are not contaminated. Treatment of range soil to kill ova is only partially successful. Changing litter can reduce infections, but treating floors with oil is not very effective. Raising different species or different ages of birds together or in close proximity is a dangerous procedure as regards parasitism. Adult turkeys, which are carriers of gapeworms, can transmit the disease to young chicks or pheasants, although older chickens are almost resistant to infection.

Treatment

Thiabendazole (Tresaderm) is currently approved for use only in pheasants and is effective when administered in the feed. Continuous medication of pen-reared birds has been recommended, but is not economical. Several other compounds have been shown effective against S. trachea under experimental conditions. Methyl 5-benzoyl-2-benzimidazole was 100% efficacious when fed prophylactically to turkey poults. 5-isopropoxycarbonylamino-2-(4-thizolyl)-benzimidazole was found to be more efficacious than thiabendazole or disophenol. The level of control with three treatments of cambendazole on days 3-4, 6-7, and 16-17 post-infection was 94.9% in chickens and 99.1% in turkeys. Levamisole (Ergamisol), fed at a level of 0.04% for 2 days or 2 g/gal drinking water for 1 day each month, has proven effective in game birds. Fenbendazole (Panacur) at 20 mg/kg for 3-4 days is also effective.

Infectious Bursal Disease

Infectious bursal disease (also known as IBD, Gumboro Disease, Infectious Bursitis and Infectious Avian Nephrosis) is a highly contagious disease of young chickens caused by *infectious bursal disease virus* (IBDV), characterised by immunosuppression and mortality generally at 3 to 6 weeks of age. The disease was first discovered in Gumboro, Delaware in 1962. It is economically important to the poultry industry worldwide due to increased susceptibility to other diseases and negative interference with effective vaccination. In recent years, very virulent strains of IBDV (vvIBDV), causing severe mortality in chicken, have emerged in Europe, Latin America, South-East Asia, Africa and the Middle East. Infection is via the oro-faecal route, with affected bird excreting high levels of the virus for approximately 2 weeks after infection.

IBDV is a double stranded RNA virus that has a bi-segmented genome and belongs to the genus *Avibirnavirus* of family *Birnaviridae*. There are two distinct serotypes of the virus, but only serotype 1 viruses cause disease in poultry. At least six antigenic subtypes of IBDV serotype 1 have been identified by *in vitro* cross-neutralisation assay. Viruses belonging to one of these antigenic subtypes are commonly known as variants, which were reported to break through high levels of maternal antibodies in commercial flocks, causing up to 60 to 100 percent mortality rates in chickens. With the advent of highly sensitive molecular techniques, such as reverse transcription polymerase chain reaction (RT-PCR) and restriction fragment length polymorphism (RFLP), it became possible to detect the vvIBDV, to differentiate IBDV strains, and to use such information in studying the molecular epidemiology of the virus.

IBDV genome consists of two segments, A and B, which are enclosed within a nonenveloped icosahedral capsid. The genome segment B (2.9 kb) encodes VP1, the putative viral RNA polymerase. The larger segment A (3.2 kb) encodes viral proteins VP2, VP3, VP4, and VP5. Among them, VP2 protein contains important neutralising antigenic sites and elicits protective immune response and most of the amino acid (AA) changes between antigenically different IBDVs are clustered in the hypervariable region of VP2. Thus, this hypervariable region of VP2 is the obvious target for the molecular techniques applied for IBDV detection and strain variation studies.

Viral Structure

The IBDV capsid protein exhibits structural domains that show homology to those of the capsid proteins of some positive-sense single-stranded RNA viruses, such as the nodaviruses and tetraviruses, as well as the T=13 capsid shell protein of the *Reoviridae*. The T=13 shell of the IBDV capsid is formed by trimers of VP2, a protein generated by removal of the C-terminal domain from its precursor, pVP2. The trimming of pVP2 is performed on immature particles as part of the maturation process. The other major structural protein, VP3, is a multifunctional component lying under the T=13 shell that influences the inherent structural polymorphism of pVP2. The virus-encoded RNA-dependent RNA polymerase, VP1, is incorporated into the capsid through its association with VP3. VP3 also interacts extensively with the viral dsRNA genome.

Pathogenesis

The virus is attracted to lymphoid cells and especially those of B-lymphocyte origins. Young birds at around two to eight weeks of age that have highly active bursa of Fabricius are more susceptible to disease. Birds over eight weeks are resistant to challenge and will not show clinical signs unless infected by highly virulent strains.

After ingestion, the virus destroys the lymphoid follicles in the bursa of Fabricius as well as the circulating B-cells in the secondary lymphoid tissues such as GALT (gut-associated lymphoid tissue),

CALT (conjuntiva), BALT (Bronchial) caecal tonsils, Harderian gland, etc. Acute disease and death is due to the necrotising effect of these viruses on the host tissue. If the bird survives and recovers from this phase of the disease, it remains immunocompromised which means it is more susceptible to other diseases.

Clinical Signs

In the acute form birds are depressed, debilitated and dehydrated. They produce watery diarrhea and have swollen, bloodstained vent. It is common for the birds to be recumbent and show a ruffling of the feathers.

Mortality rates vary with virulence of the strain involved, the challenge dose as well as the flock's ability to mount an effective immune response. Infection with less virulent strains may not show overt clinical signs but the birds may have fibrotic or cystic bursa of Fabricus that has atrophied prematurely (before six months of age) and may die of infections by agents that would not usually cause disease in immunocompetent birds.

Diagnosis

A preliminary diagnosis can usually be made based on flock history, clinical signs and *post-mortem* (necropsy) examinations. However, definitive diagnosis can only be achieved by the specific detection and/or isolation and characterisation of IBDV. Immunofluorescence or immunohistochemistry tests, based on anti-IBDV labelled antibodies, or insitu hybridisation, based on labelled complementary cDNA sequence probe, are useful for the specific detection of IBDV in infected tissues.

RT-PCR (as mentioned above) was designed for the detection of IBDV genome, such as VP1 coding gene, with the possibility of PCR product sequences be determined for genetically comparing isolates and producing phylogenetic trees. Serological tests such as agar gel precipitation and ELISA, for detecting antibodies, are used for monitoring vaccine responses and might be an additional information of infection for unvaccinated flocks.

Necropsy examination will usually show changes in the bursa of Fabricius such as swelling, oedema, haemorrhage, the presence of a creamy transudate and eventually, atrophy. Pathological changes, especially haemorrhages, may also be seen in the muscle, intestines, kidney and spleen.

Treatment & Control

Vaccination in the face of outbreak will not be effective, therefore no treatment is available.

Passive immunity protects against disease, as does previous infection with avirulent strains. In broiler farms, breeder flocks are immunised against IBD so that they would confer protective antibodies to their progenies, which would be slaughtered for consumption before their passive immunity wears out. The vaccines themselves can cause immunosuppression and damage to the bursa of fabricus. Appropriate hygiene measures are essential for prevention and control as the virus can survive for long periods in both housing and water.

Infectious Bursal Disease

Etiology and Transmission

Infectious bursal disease is caused by a birnavirus (IBDV) that is most readily isolated from the bursa of Fabricius but may be isolated from other organs. It is shed in the feces and transferred from house to house by fomites. It is very stable and difficult to eradicate from premises.

IBDV may be isolated in 8 to 11 day old, antibody-free chicken embryos with inocula from birds in the early stages of disease. The chorioallantoic membrane is more sensitive to inoculation than is the allantoic sac. IBDV also may be isolated in cell cultures derived from the cloacal bursa and established cell lines, and some strains may be isolated in chicken-embryo fibroblasts. Cell-culture-adapted strains of IBDV produce a cytopathic effect and may be used for quantitative serologic tests. Two serotypes of IBDV have been identified; within them, antigenic variation between strains is considerable. Serotype 2 infects chickens and turkeys but does not cause clinical disease or immunosuppression.

"Variant" strains of IBDV, which have major antigenic differences from the "standard" strains, cause immunosuppression but not clinical disease in older chickens.

Clinical Findings

Infectious bursal disease is highly contagious; results of infection depend on age and breed of chicken and virulence of the virus. Infections may be subclinical or clinical. Infections before 3 wk of age are usually subclinical. Chickens are most susceptible to clinical disease at 3-6 wk, but severe infections have occurred in Leghorn chickens up to 18 wk old.

Early subclinical infections are the most important form of the disease because of economic losses. They cause severe, long-lasting immunosuppression due to destruction of immature lymphocytes in the bursa of Fabricius, thymus, and spleen. The humoral (B cell) immune response is most severely affected; the cell-mediated (T cell) immune response is affected to a lesser extent. Chickens immunosuppressed by early IBDV infections do not respond well to vaccination and are predisposed to infections with normally nonpathogenic viruses and bacteria. Common diseases are usually exacerbated by IBDV infections. Subclinical infections by the "variant" strains occur in immature birds, and severe longterm immunosuppression and bursal atrophy result from early infections.

In clinical infections, onset of the disease is sudden after an incubation of 3-4 days. Chickens exhibit severe prostration, incoordination, watery diarrhea, soiled vent feathers, vent picking, and inflammation of the cloaca. Losses range to >20%. Recovery occurs in <1 wk, and broiler weight gain is delayed by 3-5 days. The presence of maternal antibody will modify the clinical course of the disease. Virulence of field strains of the virus varies considerably. Very virulent (vv) strains of the virus that cause high mortality and morbidity were detected first in Europe. These spread throughout the Old World in the last decade and in 1999 were in South America. The vv strains have not been detected in the USA.

Lesions

At necropsy, the cloacal bursa is swollen, edematous, yellowish, and occasionally hemorrhagic, especially in birds that have died of the disease. Congestion and hemorrhage of the pectoral, thigh, and leg muscles is common. Chickens recovered from IBDV infections have small, atrophied, cloacal bursas due to the destruction and lack of regeneration of the bursal follicles.

Control

There is no treatment. Depopulation and rigorous disinfection of contaminated farms have achieved limited success. Live vaccines of chick-embryo or cell-culture origin and of varying virulence can be administered by eye drop, drinking water, or SC routes at 1-21 days of age. The immune response can be altered by maternal antibody, and the more virulent vaccine strains can override higher levels of antibody.

High levels of maternal antibody during early brooding of chicks in broiler flocks (and in some commercial layer operations) can minimise early infection, subsequent immunosuppression, or both. Breeder flocks should be vaccinated one or more times during the growing period, first with a live vaccine and again just before egg production with an oil-adjuvanted, inactivated vaccine. Inactivated vaccines of chick-embryo, bursa, or cell-culture origin are available. The latter vaccines induce higher, more uniform, and more persistent levels of antibody than do live vaccines. The immune status of breeder flocks should be monitored periodically with a quantitative serologic test such as virus neutralisation or ELISA. If antibody levels fall, hens should be revaccinated to maintain adequate immunity in the progeny.

Bloodborne Organisms

Avian blood may contain various disease agents including viruses, bacteria, rickettsiae, protozoa, microfilariae, and rarely fungi. Except for viruses, these organisms often can be identified by microscopic examination of wet mounts, buffy coat, or blood smears; appropriate culturing techniques; or subinoculation of blood into susceptible birds. Microscopically, some are within blood cells (Plasmodium, Haemoproteus, Leucocytozoon, Atoxoplasma, Hepatocystis, Babesia, Aegyptianella), while others are free in the plasma (Trypanosoma, microfilariae, bacteria, spirochetes). None lives exclusively in the blood; most are found in tissues but are present in blood during part of their life cycle. Some, such as microfilariae and Plasmodium, may have a periodicity when numbers or stages of parasites are present at different times. In such cases, examining multiple smears at intervals will increase the likelihood of obtaining a diagnosis. Seasonal variations in infection rates relate to the activity of arthropod vectors. When possible, tissue cytology is also a useful adjunct to examination of blood. Several bloodborne organisms are either uncommon or not associated with clinical disease. However, weakened or injured raptors infected with hemoprotozoa had higher mortality and delayed recovery compared with uninfected birds. Routine examination for bloodborne organisms should be included in the clinical and diagnostic procedures for any ill bird.

Thin blood smears should be made with blood directly from the bird if possible. Anticoagulants, storage, and cooling of the blood can distort protozoan morphology and introduce artifacts. A small drop of blood can be collected using a syringe and needle, or by selecting a small vessel in the wing web and, after cleaning the site thoroughly with alcohol and letting it dry, puncturing the vessel with a lancet so that a small drop of blood wells up from the wound. The drop should be picked up without touching the skin and spread on a clean glass slide at a 30° angle to make a thin smear. A good quality Romanowsky-type stain that gives good polychromatic coloration (eg, Giemsa stain) should be used. At least 200 oil-immersion fields (~20,000 RBC) for single smears or 100 for multiple smears from the same bird should be examined. Leucocytozoon and microfilariae are found around the periphery of smears and can be easily seen on low-power magnification.

Bloodborne organisms in plasma or WBC are concentrated in the buffy coat. A diamond-tipped pencil can be used to cut the microhematocrit tube just below the buffy coat above the packed RBC. The buffy coat should be expressed from the cut end with a small amount of plasma to make a suspension, and a thin smear prepared. Stained buffy coat smears are recommended for detecting bacteremia, spirochetes, and chronic Leucocytozoon, Trypanosoma, or Atoxoplasma infections. An excellent technique for identifying low numbers of motile organisms such as spirochetes and microfilariae is direct examination of the buffy coat by darkfield or phase contrast microscopy. The buffy coat and all of the plasma should be expressed onto a glass slide, and covered with a coverglass, which is depressed slightly to spread the buffy coat. The buffy coat/plasma interface should be examined with darkfield or reduced light microscopy to detect motile organisms.

Plasmodium infections can be determined by subinoculation. Ideally, birds of the same or a known susceptible avian species should be used, but this is often not practical. In general, canaries are used for detecting passerine infections, and turkeys are susceptible to most plasmodia that infect gallinaceous birds. Parasites remain viable in blood stored at 32°F (in ice) for at least 7 days. Inoculation IV is preferred and will result in earlier parasitemia, but any parenteral route can be used. Recipients should be examined twice weekly for a minimum of 4 wk if exposed IV; longer times are needed if other routes of inoculation are used. Spirochete, Aegyptianella, and bacterial infections can also be detected by subinoculation of infectious blood; bacteria can usually be identified by blood culture.

To make a diagnosis of infection with an intracellular blood protozoan on a thin blood film, it first should be determined that the "parasites" in question are neither normal nor artifact. The following should then be determined: the host cell and whether it is normal or deformed beyond identification, whether pigment granules are present or absent, and whether merogony is occurring. Identification of an organism beyond genus (or subgenus in the case of Plasmodium spp) is difficult and usually unnecessary for clinical purposes.

Aegyptianellosis

Aegyptianellosis is an acute, tickborne, febrile disease caused by Aegyptianella spp, a rickettsia in the family Anaplasmataceae. Infection of avian species, including chickens, turkeys, guineafowl, quail, pigeons, crows, waterfowl, ratites, passerines, and psittacines has been described. Ticks, especially Argas spp, transmit the organism; infection can also be reproduced by blood inoculation. Organisms appear as single or multiple, round, "signet-ring" (0.5-4 μm) or irregular oval bodies in RBC often lateral to the nucleus. Infections are most common in tropical and subtropical areas of Africa, Asia, and Europe; infection of wild turkeys in Texas has also been reported.

In endemic areas, infection is mild or asymptomatic. Ruffled feathers, anorexia, droopiness, diarrhea, fever, jaundice, and high mortality in younger birds occur in introduced or otherwise susceptible birds. Anaemia, which can lead to right heart failure and ascites, enlargement of the liver and spleen, enlarged discoloured kidneys, and pinpoint serosal hemorrhages are seen. Infestation with larval argasid ticks and Borrelia infection (spirochetosis, *Avian Spirochetosis: Introduction*) may accompany the disease.

Tetracyclines, especially doxycycline, are effective in controlling the disease and eliminating the organism from chronically infected birds. Tick control is an important adjunct to treatment.

Atoxoplasmosis (Isosporosis, Lankesterellosis)

Atoxoplasma are pale-staining, nonpigmented, oval, intracytoplasmic bodies within mononuclear cells currently thought to be lymphocytes. Usually, cells contain a single parasite, but multiple organisms can be seen in severe, acute infections. Presence of the protozoan causes the nucleus to curve around it giving the appearance that the organism is located within an indentation of the nucleus. At least 2 different genera of coccidian protozoa (Isospora, Lankesterella) have merozoites in the lymphocytes that are indistinguishable from each other and have been called Atoxoplasma. Passerine birds, especially canaries, finches, sparrows, and species of the Sturnidae family (starlings, mynahs) are affected by both protozoa. Poultry are not known to be affected.

Isospora has a direct life cycle that includes an extra-intestinal, systemic phase in some species. Merogony occurs in the intestine and oocysts are passed in the feces. The systemic part of the life cycle was initially not recognised, leading to the description of the intestinal stages and oocysts as Isospora serini. Transmission is faecal-oral via ingestion of oocysts in droppings from infected birds. Infected canaries can shed oocysts for at least 2 yr. Most species of avian Isospora do not have extra-intestinal stages. In canaries, I serini has a systemic phase while I canaria infects only the intestinal tract.

Lankesterella has stages in the blood indistinguishable from those caused by systemic Isospora spp, but merogony occurs in tissues other than the intestine, especially the lungs. The life cycle is indirect. Bloodsucking arthropods, particularly mites, become infected during feeding and transmit the protozoan when it refeeds on a susceptible bird.

Signs include listlessness, diarrhea, and anorexia. Mortality can be high (up to 80%) in young birds. In acutely affected birds, there is marked hepatomegaly and splenomegaly, often with multifocal necrosis. The enlarged liver and gallbladder can be seen through the abdominal wall, especially if it is moistened with alcohol, which provides the basis for the common name black spot disease. High numbers of parasites infecting lymphocytes are present in blood and organ impression smears. Nearly spherical oocysts averaging 19×21 µm are present in droppings of canaries infected with Isospora. Oocysts of I serini need to be distinguished from those of I canaria, which are slightly larger and more oval.

Diagnosis is difficult in chronically infected older birds. Very few parasites are present in blood and tissues, and oocysts are shed intermittently, although sometimes in high numbers. Buffy coat and organ smears are preferred. Negative findings should not be interpreted to mean that infection is not present. Hepatic and splenic enlargement persists because of infiltrations with high numbers of large lymphoid cells that serve as host cells for the parasite. Histopathologically, organisms are difficult to find and identify. Lesions may be mistaken for lymphosarcoma.

There is no known effective treatment. Anticoccidial drugs do not affect parasites in the tissues. Use of antimalarial drugs has been suggested. Good management procedures, including prevention of exposure to mites, isolation of age groups, and scrupulous cleanliness (particularly daily cleaning before oocysts sporulate) help control the disease. Disinfectants have little effect on oocysts.

Filariasis

Microfilariae are commonly found in the blood of wild birds but are rare to absent in poultry except in southeast Asia where infections in chickens and waterfowl occur. A high percentage of imported cockatiels have microfilariae. At least 16 genera of filarids are found in avian species. All have an indirect life cycle with bloodsucking insects (eg, lice, mosquitos, midges) serving as intermediate hosts. Adults are relatively short lived and mature in body cavities, including the eye and ventricles of the brain, respiratory system, cardiovascular system, or connective tissues; some produce characteristic subcutaneous nodules. In contrast, microfilariae are long lived and may be numerous in the skin as well as in the circulation. Increased numbers of microfilariae have been seen in stressed individuals, but they rarely cause clinical disease or mortality. A possible exception is infection of emus with Chandlerella, a common filarid of the brain of free-living grackles. Parasites apparently do not produce microfilariae iemus. Affected emus show signs of CNS disease. Treatment with ivermectin, levamisole, or injection of nodules with 0.5% potassium permanganate solution, and surgical removal of adults have been used.

Haemoproteus Infection

Infections with Haemoproteus spp are common in nondomestic birds. Pigeons and doves are frequently infected. Species are found in free-living ducks, quail, and turkeys but are rare to absent in commercial flocks probably because of very specific feeding habits of Culicoides spp and hippoboscid flies, the invertebrate vectors. In free-living bird populations, females are more frequently infected than males. Until recently, Haemoproteus was considered relatively innocuous and of little clinical significance. Fatal infections can occur because of extensive widespread necrosis accompanying development of large exoerythrocytic megalomeronts in muscle, heart, liver, and lung. Mortality as high as 78% has occurred in bobwhite quail infected with Isospora lophortyx. Similar meronts and lesions have been reported previously in cases of "aberrant leucocytozoonosis" and arthrocystosis. The diagnostic presence of large, pigmented gametocytes in mature RBC that often partially or completely encircle the nucleus without merogony can follow or occur simultaneously with systemic involvement. Sudden death without clinical signs or a prolonged course of weakness, lameness, dyspnea, lethargy, poor growth, and anaemia may be seen. Little is known about effective treatment, although antimalarial drugs may be tried. Chloroquine (5 mg/kg) and buparvaquone (2.5 mg/kg) have been reported to be effective in treating pigeons; diminazene and quinapyramine were either ineffective or toxic. Measures to control invertebrate hosts should help prevent heavy infections.

Leucocytozoonosis

Infections with Leucocytozoon spp range from subclinical to fatal. Mortality may approach 100% but varies greatly with species and strain of parasite, host species, degree of exposure, and other factors. Acute outbreaks of leucocytozoonosis have been reported in chickens (Asia, Africa), turkeys (North America), waterfowl (North America, Europe), and a number of free-living and captive avian species throughout the world. Species in domestic birds include L simondi in waterfowl; L smithi in turkeys; and L caulleryi, L sabrazesi, L andrewsi, and L schoutedeni in chickens. L caulleryi can be highly pathogenic, causing a lethal hemorrhagic disease of chickens in southeast Asia. Numerous Leucocytozoon spp infect nondomestic birds (eg, blood smears from raptors often contain gametocytes). Clinical disease and mortality result from anaemia caused by antierythrocytic factors produced by the parasite, high numbers of the large gametocytes blocking pulmonary capillaries, or parasites invading the endothelium of vessels in vital tissues (brain, heart, etc.) where they form megalomeronts that occlude vessels and result in multifocal necrosis.

Wild birds are reservoirs in some areas and are responsible for initiating infection in young birds each year. Parasitemia often increases dramatically in late April and early May (called spring rise), just before arthropod vectors, black flies (Simulium spp), or biting midges (Culicoides spp) increase. Ducks that have recovered from infection with L simondi relapse when light cycles are manipulated to increase egg production. Increased levels of prolactin have been suggested as a possible cause.

Acute disease is seen more often in the young when they have high parasitemia and when black flies or biting midges are most abundant. Subacute or chronic disease is seen in the young outside fly season and in older birds at any season; parasitemia is usually low. Recovered birds remain carriers and serve as a reservoir for young, susceptible birds.

Clinical Findings, Lesions, and Diagnosis

Acutely affected birds are listless and have anaemia, leukocytosis, tachypnea, anorexia, diarrhea with green droppings, and often CNS signs. Egg production is impaired in laying chickens infected with L caulleryi. Signs are evident ~1 wk after infection and coincide with the onset of parasitemia. Visibly affected birds die after 7-10 days or may recover with sequelae of poor growth and egg production. Hemorrhages, splenomegaly, and hepatomegaly are seen. Grossly visible white dots in affected organs are megalomeronts.

In thin blood smears, gametocytes may be seen along the edges and tail of the smear. Leucocytozoon is identified by large gametocytes that lack pigment and distort the host cell (RBC or WBC), making it no longer identifiable. Shape of gametocytes varies with the species— some are elongated with long tapering extremities, while others are round. Serology may detect prior infection.

Treatment and Control

Treatment usually is not effective. Preventive medication with combined pyrimethamine (1 ppm) and sulfadimethoxine (10 ppm) combined in the feed controls L caulleryi; clopidol (0.0125-0.025%) controls L smithi. Measures to control invertebrate vectors are helpful. Humoral immunity resulting from vaccination will protect against L caulleryi infection.

Plasmodium Infection

Plasmodium spp, which often are not host-specific, infect a wide variety of domestic and wild birds in most areas of the world and can cause high losses. P gallinaceum infects chickens in Asia and Africa and causes low mortality in indigenous chickens but rates may be as high as 80-90% in commercial birds. P juxtanucleare infects chickens in Asia, Africa, and South America; most infections are mild or asymptomatic. P durae infects turkeys and gallinaceous birds other than chickens in Africa; mortality in turkeys can approach 100%. Clinical malaria has not been reported from poultry in North America, but indigenous wild turkeys can become infected with at least 4 different Plasmodium species. Asymptomatic infections in endemic or introduced birds can be spread via mosquitos and cause fatal disease in introduced (eg, zoo penguins) or resident (eg, Hawaiian avifauna) birds, respectively. Invertebrate hosts are ornithophilic mosquitos, usually Culex, Culiseta, or Aedes spp.

Clinical Findings, Lesions, and Diagnosis

Infection with Plasmodium spp may be nonclinical or cause illness characterised by weakness, lassitude, dyspnea, anaemia, abdominal distention, increased right heart weight, ocular hemorrhage, and death. Death results from severe anaemia or blockage of capillaries in the brain or other vital organs by exoerythrocytic meronts in endothelial cells. Liver and spleen are markedly enlarged and often discoloured (dark brown to black). Pigmented parasites including meronts are found in both immature and mture RBC. Infrequently, parasites are found in thrombocytes and WBC. In birds that die acutely, organisms may be sparse or absent in blood, but numerous meronts can be found in capillaries by examining squash or impression smears of brain, lung, liver, and spleen. Serologic and molecular diagnostic methods are under development but are not yet available for general use. Serology can detect infection when parasites are too few to be identified in blood smears.

Treatment and Control

Chemotherapy is variably effective in treating infected birds or flocks. Chloroquine (5-10 mg/kg) potentiated with primaquine (0.3 mg/kg), or chloroquine in drinking water (250 mg/120 mL) has been used. Grape or orange juice can disguise chloroquine's bitterness. Other antimalarial drugs have been used with success; quinacrine at 1.6 mg/kg/day for 5 days was successful for treating an infected peacock. Treatment with a combination of sulfamonomethoxine and sulfachloropyrazine is effective; halofuginone can be used for chemoprophylaxis in endemic areas. Persistent parasitemia or relapse may occur during and after treatment. Treatments should be evaluated on prevention of mortality and improvement of clinical disease. Birds that survive initial infection are generally refractory to subsequent infections. Prevention of exposure to mosquitos is a useful adjunct. Parasite development is reduced in mosquitos that survive previous infection with Bacillus thuringiensis *israelensis*.

Other Bloodborne Organisms

Trypanosomes have been described in several avian species but rarely if ever cause clinical disease. They are more commonly identified in organ smears, especially bone marrow, than in peripheral blood, and can be cultured. Invertebrate hosts are thought to be any of several bloodsucking insects. Treatment is not warranted.

Borreliae are tickborne (Argas spp) spirochetes that can cause fatal systemic disease. Tetracyclines, penicillin, and tick control are used for prevention and treatment.

Small, punctate, or rarely ring-shaped, rickettsia-like basophilic bodies resembling Pirhemocyton, an organism that infects reptiles, are frequently seen in avian erythrocytes. Their identity and significance are unknown. They tend to be smaller and morphologically distinct from Aegyptianella.

Babesia spp are uncommon, nonpigmented, pyriform-shaped, erythrocytic protozoan parasites of birds. Natural infections of penguins, falcons, cranes, and several Asian avian species occur. Ticks are considered to be the invertebrate hosts. V, X, or fan shapes characterise dividing forms. Nothing is known of their significance, treatment, or control.

Haemogregarina and Hepatozoon are protozoan parasites that are infrequently identified in birds. Both produce relatively large, nonpigmented, elongated gametocytes that can be found in RBC and WBC respectively. Gametocytes of Haemogregarina resemble gametocytes of Haemoproteus but lack pigment and are smaller, rarely if ever extending around or encircling the nucleus. Gametocytes of Hepatozoon are elongated with rounded ends and usually not located within an indentation of the nucleus, whereas Atoxoplasma is oval and partially encircled by the nucleus.

Zoites of other sporozoa (eg, Toxoplasma, Sarcocystis) and organisms normally in the digestive tract (eg, trichomonads, coccidia, histomonads) may be transiently found in blood. The latter often also produce liver lesions.

Chapter 6

Chicken Anaemia Virus Infection

Chicken Infectious Anaemia, Blue Wing Disease, Anaemia Dermatitis Syndrome, Hemorrhagic Aplastic Anaemia Syndrome

Chicken anaemia virus (CAV), a 25 nm, nonenveloped, icosahedral virus with a single-stranded, circular DNA genome, is the only member of the genus Gyrovirus of the Circoviridae family. The genome codes for 3 viral proteins (VP). VP1 is the capsid protein, but VP2 may be needed as a scaffold protein to allow proper folding of VP1. VP3, or apoptin, is a nonstructural protein that induces apoptosis in infected cells. CAV infects only chickens, although antibodies have been detected in Japanese quail. The virus is present worldwide based on serology and virus isolation. The disease, chicken infectious anaemia, has been described in most countries where chickens are raised commercially.

Horizontal transmission of CAV is by the faecal-oral route and perhaps by the respiratory route. Vertical transmission occurs when seronegative hens become infected and continues until neutralising antibodies develop. Chicks hatched from these eggs are viremic, and CAV can rapidly spread horizontally from these chicks to susceptible, maternal antibody-negative hatchmates. Roosters shedding CAV in the semen are another source of vertical transmission. Vaccination of seronegative flocks prior to the onset of egg production is recommended to prevent vertical transmission.

Maternal antibody-negative chicks are susceptible to infection and disease until 1-2 wk of age. In contrast, maternal antibody-positive chicks are protected from disease and probably from infection. Age resistance to clinical disease, but not infection, begins at approximately 1 wk of age. The age resistance can be overcome by coinfection of CAV with immunosuppressive agents such as infectious bursal disease virus (*Infectious Bursal Disease: Introduction*), Marek's disease herpesvirus (*Marek's Disease*), and reticuloendotheliosis virus (*Reticuloendotheliosis*).

Many SPF flocks developed antibodies to CAV during or after the onset of sexual development. Spread of infection by CAV-contaminated embryo- or cell-culture-derived vaccines is possible.

When day-old susceptible chicks are inoculated IM with CAV, viraemia occurs within 24 hr. Virus can be recovered from most organs and rectal contents up to 35 days after inoculation. The principal sites of CAV replication are hemocytoblasts in the bone marrow, precursor T cells in the cortex of the thymus, and CD8 cells in the spleen. Replication in the first leads to anaemia, while replication in the latter two causes immunosuppression. Neutralising antibodies are detectable 21 days after infection and clinical, hematologic, and pathologic parametres return to normal ~35 days after infection. CAV infection has adverse effects on proliferative responses of spleen lymphocytes and on the production of interleukin. and interferons by splenocytes. Infection can cause a marked decrease in generation of antigen-specific cytotoxic T cells directed against other pathogens. In addition to T-cell defects, macrophage functions such as Fc-receptor expression, phagocytosis, and antimicrobial activity may be impaired. Subclinical, horizontally acquired infection with CAV in broiler progeny of seropositive parent flocks may be associated with impaired economic performance.

Clinical Findings

Signs of illness or adverse effects on egg production do not occur when seronegative adult chickens become infected. However, vertical transmission or infection of maternal antibody-negative chicks before 1 wk of age can cause clinical disease 12-17 days after hatching or infection. Chicks are anorectic, lethargic, depressed, and pale. PCV is low (in chicks, anaemia is defined as a PCV of d"27), and blood smears often reveal anaemia, leukopenia, or pancytopenia depending on the state of the disease. Blood may be watery and clot slowly. Mortality rates are variable but may be high with secondary complicating infections.

Lesions

Organs are pale; the thymus is generally atrophied, and the bursa of Fabricius may be small. Bone marrow is pale or yellow. Hemorrhage may be present in or under the skin, muscle, and other organs. Histologically, lymphoid cell populations are depleted in primary and secondary lymphoid organs. Granulocytic and erythrocytic compartments in the bone marrow are atrophic or hypoplastic.

Diagnosis

A tentative diagnosis is based on history, signs, and gross and histopathologic lesions. Confirmation requires detection of virus or viral DNA in the thymus or bone marrow. PCR and quantitative PCR techniques are commonly used to demonstrate the presence of CAV. Viral isolation can be used but is slow and expensive. To isolate CAV, chloroform-treated extracts of tissues are inoculated in MDCC-MSB1 or MDCC-147 cultures (a lymphoblastoid cell line derived from Marek's disease tumour) or into susceptible, immunocompromised (antigen- and antibody-negative), day-old chicks. Commercial ELISA kits are available to detect serum antibodies to CAV and can be used to identify breeder flocks that are seronegative prior to egg production and to monitor the efficacy of vaccination.

Treatment and Prevention

There is no specific treatment. Secondary bacterial infections may be treated with antibiotics. Live vaccines are available for vaccination of antibody-negative breeder flocks prior to the start of egg production. Administration is by injection or by addition to the drinking water depending on the type of vaccine available in individual countries. In some areas, transfer of litter to noncontaminated premises and the addition of crude homogenates of tissues from affected chickens to the drinking water have been used to ensure infection and seroconversion of parent flocks before they begin to lay, thereby diminishing the risk of egg transmission. However, these procedures are risky and not recommended. Because of the synergism between CAV and other immunosuppressive viruses, control of the latter is also important.

At present, there is no vaccine available to prevent subclinical losses in broilers.

Dissecting Aneurysm

Dissecting aneurysm is a fatal disease of turkeys characterised by sudden death of rapidly growing birds with massive internal hemorrhage resulting from rupture of aneurysms formed in various parts of the vascular system. The frequency with which the posterior aorta is affected has given rise to the term "aortic rupture." The disease has been reported in North America, Europe, and Israel. Most breeds of turkeys are susceptible, and the largest and most rapidly growing males, 8-24 wk old, are affected most often; females are also affected but at a lower incidence.

Etiology

The cause is unknown. Probably several factors contribute to the development of fatal cases. For the disease to occur, birds must be fed and managed in such a way that they are growing rapidly, and they must have a genetic susceptibility. A prolonged lipemia generally develops during the period of rapid growth, and the period of greatest mortality typically corresponds to a sharp rise in blood pressure, with dissecting aneurysms developing at the site of arteriosclerotic plaques. The lipemia may result from a high dietary intake of fat or from the effects of hormonal factors, such as high dietary concentrations of estrogens. Although â-aminopropionitrile, the toxic agent in Lathyrus odouratus, is capable of producing the disease, there is no evidence that this or other nitriles are responsible for dissecting aneurysms in turkeys under natural conditions. The enzyme lysyloxidase, isolated from turkey aortas and active on tropelaston and collagen cross-linking, was found to be much lower in males than females; this may be a factor in the development of spontaneous aortic aneurysms in male turkeys.

Clinical Findings

Affected birds that had shown no premonitory signs are found dead with marked pallor of the head and neck. Occasionally, a caretaker observes an apparently healthy bird die within a few minutes. The incidence is usually <1% but may be as great as 10%. Formerly, when male turkeys were implanted with stilbestrol, the incidence was as high as 20%.

Lesions

The carcass is markedly anaemic with large quantities of clotted blood in the peritoneal cavity and over the kidneys, or in the pericardial sac. The rupture in the ventral wall of the posterior aorta at about the position of the testes, or in the cardiac atrium, can be located readily by carefully washing away the blood clot. The aortic lumen may contain an organised, adherent thrombus at the site of rupture.

Ruptures in smaller blood vessels are more difficult to locate. Almost always, an intimal thickening or a large, fibrous plaque is present in the region of the rupture. The tunicas intima and media are thrown into deep folds and separated from the tunica adventitia. Marked accumulation of lipids in the thickened intima and in the fibrous plaques can be identified by stains. Fibres of the tunica media may show degenerative changes and infiltration with heterophils and macrophages.

Diagnosis

The diagnosis is made by finding large clots of blood in the coelomic cavity (aortic rupture) or within the pericardial sac (auricular rupture) of rapidly growing male turkeys. The condition should be differentiated from hypertensive angiopathy (*Perirenal Hemorrhage Syndrome of Turkeys: Introduction*), which is also seen in rapidly growing turkeys. In hypertensive angiopathy, the major lesions include pulmonary edema and supcapsular perirenal hemorrhage.

Treatment, Control, and Prevention

There is no known treatment. Coagulants and vitamin K are useless because there is no defect in the clotting mechanism. Losses sometimes may be reduced during the critical period between 16 and 23 wk of age by limiting feed intake or slowing growth rate by reducing the energy level of the diet. High-fat diets should not be fed during this period. Some studies have indicated that the incidence of aortic rupture can be reduced by adding copper at 125-250 ppm to the diet from at least 4 wk of age until market.

Inclusion Body Hepatitis Hydropericardium Syndrome

Hepatitis Hydropericardium

Adenoviruses are widespread throughout all avian species. Studies have demonstrated the presence of antibodies in healthy poultry, and viruses have been isolated from normal birds. Despite their widespread distribution, the majority of adenoviruses cause no or only mild disease; however, some are associated with specific clinical conditions. Avian adenoviruses (AAV) in chickens are the etiologic agents of 2 important diseases known as inclusion body hepatitis (IBH) and hydropericardium syndrome (HP). Although in some cases each condition is observed separately, during the last decade the 2 conditions have been frequently observed as a single entity; therefore, the name hepatitis hydropericardium has been widely used to describe the pathologic condition. The syndrome is an acute disease of young chickens associated with anaemia, hemorrhagic disorders, and hydropericardium. It is a common disease in several countries, where broilers are severely affected, resulting in high mortality rates.

Etiology, Transmission, and Pathogenesis

The AAV of group I are the etiologic agents of this condition. Although there are 12 different serotypes of AAV, the most common viruses isolated in cases of IBH/HP belong to serotypes 4 and 8. These AAV are capable of producing the disease without the immunosuppressive effects of associated viruses such as infectious bursal disease (IBDV, *Infectious Bursal Disease: Introduction*) or other immunosuppressive agents. However, the association with immunosuppressive viruses such as IBDV and chicken anaemia virus (CAV, *Chicken Anaemia Virus Infection: Introduction*) will result in a more severe disease.

Horizontal and vertical transmission play an important role in IBH/HP. Vertical transmission has been described in progeny from breeder flocks infected with AAV serotypes 4 and 8. Horizontal transmission has also been demonstrated; young chicks in contact with infected chicks can die of peracute IBH/HP. Chicks and young chickens are commonly affected. Infection with some strains of AAV may result in minimal hepatic disease; however, if birds have been infected with immunosuppressive viruses (IBD, CAV, Marek's disease), the clinical disease becomes evident.

Clinical Findings, Lesions, and Diagnosis

Sudden mortality usually is seen in chickens <6 wk old and as young as 4 days of age. Mortality normally ranges from 2-40%, especially when birds are <3 wk of age. However, there have been outbreaks in which mortality has reached 80%. Mortality rates also vary depending on the pathogenicity of the virus and infection with other viral or bacterial agents. Signs associated with diseases caused by other pathogens (eg, bacteria, fungi, or viruses) commonly occur if birds are immunosuppressed.

Flocks of 3 to 5 wk old broilers with HP may not show specific clinical signs, but abrupt onset of mortality, lethargy, huddling with ruffled feathers, and yellow, mucoid droppings may be seen. The duration of the infection usually ranges from 9-14 days with morbidity of 10-30% and a daily mortality of 3-5%. Gross lesions include up to 10 mL of a straw-coloured transudate in the pericardial sac, generalised congestion, and an enlarged, pale, friable liver. Histopathologic lesions include myocardial edema in the heart with degeneration, necrosis, and mild mononuclear cell infiltration. Basophilic intranuclear inclusion bodies may be present in the liver. A tentative diagnosis is based on typical microscopic findings and confirmed by isolating adenoviruses from the liver. Serology, restriction enzyme analysis and PCR are used to classify adenoviruses isolated from clinical cases. This information is used for epidemiologic studies.

Treatment and Prevention

As with many other viral diseases, there is no treatment. Antibiotics may help prevent secondary bacterial infections. Sulfonamides are contraindicated if evidence of hematologic disease or immunosuppression is seen.

Vaccines against IBH/HP are not commercially available in the USA; however, in other countries both live and inactivated vaccines are used to control the syndrome. The AAV serotypes most frequently used to prepare commercial vaccines are serotypes 4 and 8. Primary breeders with stringent biosecurity practices sometimes use autogenous inactivated vaccines to ensure the transfer of maternal immunity from breeding flocks to their progeny.

In Australia, a live vaccine given via drinking water was developed for breeders between 10-14 wk of age. In other countries, including Mexico, Pakistan, and Peru, inactivated vaccines are routinely used to vaccinate breeders and broilers.

When breeders are properly vaccinated, antibodies generated by the vaccine are transmitted to the progeny, providing protection against field infections and clinical disease. Broilers are vaccinated at <10 days of age when their parents either do not have serotype-specific adenovirus antibodies or maternal antibody transmission is erratic due to improper vaccination procedures that result in a substantial number of unvaccinated birds.

Perirenal Hemorrhage Syndrome of Turkeys

Hypertensive Angiopathy, Sudden Death Syndrome of Turkeys

Perirenal hemorrhage syndrome (PHS) is a noninfectious cardiovascular disease usually affecting rapidly growing male turkeys

8-15 wk old characterised by sudden death, perirenal hemorrhage, and hypertrophic cardiomyopathy. Mortality is usually 0.5-2% but can be higher; there is no morbidity. Healthy, rapidly growing flocks are more likely to be affected.

The pathogenesis is unknown, but PHS is apparently unrelated to pulmonary function or hypertension. Inadequate or inappropriate cardiac response to exercise, resulting in hypotension, vasodilation, arrhythmias, and sudden death, appears most likely. Acute congestive heart failure secondary to cardiac hypertrophy has also been suggested as a potential cause. Renal hemorrhage may occur due to severe passive congestion.

Gross lesions include good to excellent body condition, food in crop and stomach, enlarged dark red to purple spleen, variable retroperitoneal hemorrhage around one or both kidneys, generalised congestion, and pulmonary edema occasionally accompanied by hemorrhage.

Cardiac hypertrophy involving the left ventricle and intraventricular septum may also be seen. Microscopic changes are consistent with gross findings; proliferative arterial and arteriolar lesions and ruptured renal veins also are often present. PHS has several characteristics in common with aortic rupture (*Dissecting Aneurysm: Introduction*) and flip-over in broilers (*Flip-over Disease: Introduction*).

Diagnosis is based on history, typical gross lesions, and absence of infectious agents. Extensive PHS lesions may resemble aortic rupture.

There is no specific treatment. Factors that decrease growth rate and activity also tend to decrease PHS. Reserpine (0.5 ppm feed) decreases PHS, but aspirin (0.005%) or increased calcium has no effect. Reserpine is not listed in the Feed Additive Compendium as approved for use in feed for turkeys. Increased room temperature and various lighting programs have also reduced PHS. Activities that increase cardiovascular stress (eg, moving birds, tilling litter, noise) should be minimised, especially between 7 and 15 wk of age. Lower ambient temperatures (55°F [13°C]), intermittent lighting, and leaving toes unclipped increase mortality from PHS.

PHS may occur in healthy commercial male turkey flocks regardless of management practices used to prevent its occurrence.

Round Heart Disease of Turkeys

Spontaneous Cardiomyopathy

Spontaneous cardiomyopathy of young turkeys is characterised by sudden death due to cardiac arrest. It has been suggested that the condition should be called spontaneous cardiomyopathy to distinguish it from round heart disease of chickens, a different syndrome that is rarely recognised today.

The exact etiology of spontaneous cardiomyopathy in turkeys is unknown. However, studies using furazolidone to produce dilated cardiomyopathy in turkeys have indicated altered membrane transport resulting in myocardial failure. Creatine kinase, glycolysis, glycogen, myofibril, Krebs cycle enzymes, fatty acid oxidation, and soluble proteins are all reduced. The calcium-transport ATPase activity of the sarcoplasmic reticulum is increased. This pattern of biochemical changes is consistent with ischemia playing a role in the pathogenesis of spontaneous cardiomyopathy in turkeys.

While most deaths occur during the brooding period, the ratio of heart weight to body weight of affected birds is increased throughout the growing period. Market body weights of affected birds are reduced an average of 3 lb (1.4 kg). Some outbreaks of the condition have been associated with hypoxia during incubation of the eggs or during transportation of poults from the hatchery to the brood farm.

Most deaths from spontaneous cardiomyopathy occur during the first 4 wk of life, with mortality peaking at 2 wk. Many poults die suddenly, but some may have ruffled feathers, drooping wings, and a general unthrifty appearance. They may show laboured, gasping breathing before death. After 3 wk of age, mortality is sporadic. Characteristically, the affected poult in the first 4 wk of life has a greatly enlarged heart due to dilatation of both ventricles, congested lungs, and a swollen liver. Ascites, anasarca, pulmonary edema, and hydropericardium may or may not be present. In older poults, enlarged hearts are due to marked hypertrophy of the ventricles in addition to dilatation. Histologically, lesions of abnormal hearts are nonspecific and include congestion, damage of the myofibrils of the cardiocytes, and focal infiltration by lymphocytes.

Generally, diagnosis is based on history and gross findings at necropsy; although an ECG can be used, it is of little practical use. Sodium and polychlorinated biphenyls or related compounds may produce similar syndromes. No treatment is available. Good brooding practices may reduce mortality. Any toxins should be eliminated. Incubation, transportation, and early brooding ventilation conditions should be reviewed.

Candidiasis

Thrush, Crop Mycosis, Sour Crop

Improving sanitation and minimising antibiotic use in poultry help reduce the incidence of candidiasis. Affected birds can be treated with copper sulfate at 0.5 mg/L of drinking water, or 0.5 mg copper sulfate per kg of feed. Vinegar is used as a treatment for candidiasis at 15 mL/L of drinking water. Chlorhexidine is used for prevention or treatment at 2.5 mL/L of drinking water. Chlorine bleach at 0.1 mL/L of drinking water may help control the infection. All of these treatments lack FDA approval.

Coccidiosis

Coccidiosis is caused by protozoa of the phylum Apicomplexa, family Eimeriidae. In poultry, most species belong to the genus Eimeria and infect various sites in the intestine. The infectious process is rapid (4-7 days) and is characterised by parasite replication in host cells with extensive damage to the intestinal mucosa. Poultry coccidia are strictly host-specific, and the different species parasitise specific parts of the intestine. Coccidia are distributed worldwide in poultry and wild birds.

Etiology

Coccidia are almost universally present in poultry-raising operations, but clinical disease occurs only after ingestion of relatively large numbers of sporulated oocysts by susceptible birds. Both clinically infected and recovered birds shed oocysts in their droppings, which contaminate feed, dust, water, litter, and soil. Oocysts may be transmitted by mechanical carriers (eg, equipment, clothing, insects, and other animals). Fresh oocysts are not infective until they sporulate; under optimal conditions (70-90°F [21-32°C] with adequate moisture and oxygen), this requires 1-2 days. The prepatent period is 4-7 days. Sporulated oocysts may survive for long periods, depending on environmental factors. Oocysts are resistant to some disinfectants commonly used around livestock but are killed by freezing or high environmental temperatures.

Pathogenicity is influenced by host genetics, nutritional factors, concurrent diseases, and species of the coccidium. Eimeria necatrix and E tenella are the most pathogenic in chickens because schizogony occurs in the lamina propria and crypts of Lieberkühn of the small intestine and ceca, respectively, and causes extensive hemorrhage. Most species develop in epithelial cells lining the villi. Protective immunity usually develops in response to moderate and continuing infection. True age-immunity does not occur, but older birds are usually more resistant than young birds because of earlier exposure to infection.

Clinical Findings

Signs range from decreased growth rate to a high percentage of visibly sick birds, severe diarrhea, and high mortality. Feed and water consumption are depressed. Weight loss, development of culls, decreased egg production, and increased mortality may accompany outbreaks. Mild infections of intestinal species, which would otherwise be classed as subclinical, may cause depigmentation. Survivors of severe infections recover in 10-14 days but may never recover lost performance.

Chickens

E tenella infections are found only in the ceca and can be recognised by accumulation of blood in the ceca and by bloody droppings. Cecal cores, which are accumulations of clotted blood, tissue debris, and oocysts, may be found in birds surviving the acute stage.

E necatrix produces major lesions in the anterior and middle portions of the small intestine. Small white spots, usually intermingled with rounded, bright- or dull-red spots of various sizes, can be seen on the serosal surface.

The white spots are diagnostic for E necatrix if clumps of large schizonts can be demonstrated microscopically. In severe cases, the intestinal wall is thickened, and the infected area dilated to 2-2.5 times the normal diametre.

The lumen may be filled with blood, mucus, and fluid. Fluid loss may result in marked dehydration. Although the damage is in the small intestine, the sexual phase of the life cycle is completed in the ceca. Oocysts of E necatrix are found only in the ceca. Due to concurrent infections, oocysts of other species may be found in the area of major lesions, misleading the diagnostician.

E acervulina, the most common infection, is characterised by numerous, whitish, oval or transverse patches in the upper half of the small intestine and may be easily distinguished on gross examination. The clinical course in a flock is usually protracted and results in poor growth, an increase in culls, and slightly increased mortality.

E brunetti is found in the lower small intestine, rectum, ceca, and cloaca. In moderate infections, the mucosa is pale and disrupted but lacking in discrete foci, and may be thickened. In severe infections, extensive coagulative necrosis and sloughing of the mucosa occurs throughout most of the small intestine.

E maxima develops in the small intestine, where it causes dilatation and thickening of the wall; petechial hemorrhage; and a reddish, orange, or pink viscous mucous exudate and fluid. The oocysts and gametocytes (particularly macrogametocytes), which are present in the lesions, are distinctly large.

E mitis is recognised as pathogenic in the lower small intestine. Lesions resemble moderate infections of E brunetti but can be distinguished by finding small, round oocysts associated with the lesion.

Turkeys

Only 4 of the 7 species of coccidia in turkeys are considered pathogenic— Eimeria adenoeides, E dispersa, E gallopavonis, and E meleagrimitis. E innocua, E meleagridis, and E subrotunda are considered nonpathogenic. Oocysts sporulate within 1-2 days after expulsion from the host; the prepatent period is 4-6 days.

E adenoeides and E gallopavonis infect the lower ileum, ceca, and rectum. The developmental stages are found in the epithelial cells of the villi and crypts. The affected portion of the intestine may be dilated and have a thickened wall. Thick, creamy material or caseous casts in the gut or excreta may contain enormous numbers of oocysts. E meleagrimitis chiefly infects the upper and mid small intestine. The lamina propria or deeper tissues may be parasitised, which may result in necrotic enteritis (*Necrotic Enteritis: Introduction*). E dispersa infects the upper small intestine and causes a creamy, mucoid enteritis that involves the entire intestine, including the ceca. Large numbers of gametocytes and oocysts are associated with the lesions.

Common signs in infected flocks include reduced feed consumption, rapid weight loss, droopiness, ruffled feathers, and severe diarrhea.

Wet droppings with mucus are common. Clinical infections are seldom seen in poults >8 wk old. Morbidity and mortality may be high.

Ducks

A large number of specific coccidia have been reported in both wild and domestic ducks, but validity of some of the descriptions is questionable. Presence of Eimeria, Wenyonella, and Tyzzeria spp has been confirmed. T perniciosa is a known pathogen that balloons the entire small intestine with mucohemorrhagic or caseous material. Eimeria spp also have been described as pathogenic. Some species of coccidia of domestic ducks are considered relatively nonpathogenic. In wild ducks, infrequent but dramatic outbreaks of coccidiosis occur in ducklings 2-4 wk old; morbidity and mortality may be high.

Geese

The most striking coccidial infection of geese is that produced by Eimeria truncata, in which the kidneys are enlarged and studded with poorly circumscribed, yellowish white streaks and spots. The tubules are dilated with masses of oocysts and urates. Mortality may be high. At least 5 other Eimeria spp have been reported to parasitise the intestine.

Diagnosis

The location in the host, appearance of lesions, and the size of oocysts are used in determining the species present. Coccidial infections are readily confirmed by demonstration of oocysts in feces or intestinal scrapings; however, the number of oocysts present has little relationship to the extent of clinical disease.

Severity of lesions as well as knowledge of flock appearance, morbidity, mortality, feed intake, growth rate, and rate of lay are important for diagnosis. Necropsy of several fresh specimens is advisable. Classical lesions of E tenella and E necatrix are pathognomonic, but infections of other species are more difficult to diagnose. Comparison of lesions and other signs with diagnostic charts allows a reasonably accurate differentiation of the coccidial species. Mixed coccidial infections are common.

A diagnosis of clinical coccidiosis is warranted if oocysts, merozoites, or schizonts are demonstrated microscopically and if lesions are severe. Subclinical coccidial infections may be unimportant, and poor performance may be caused by flock disorders.

Control

Practical methods of management cannot prevent infection. Poultry that are maintained at all times on wire floors to separate birds from droppings have fewer infections; clinical coccidiosis is seen only rarely under such circumstances. Other methods of control are vaccination or prevention with anticoccidial drugs.

Vaccination

A species-specific immunity develops after natural infection, the degree of which largely depends on the extent of infection and the number of reinfections. Protective immunity is primarily a T-cell response.

Commercial vaccines consist of low doses of live, sporulated oocysts of the various coccidial species administered at low doses to day-old chicks. Because the vaccine serves only to introduce infection, chickens are reinfected by progeny of the vaccine strain on the farm. The vaccine strains of coccidia may or may not be attenuated. The self-limiting nature of coccidiosis is used as a form of attenuation for some vaccines, rather than biological attenuation.

Layers and breeders that are maintained on floor litter must have protective immunity. Often, they are given a suboptimal dosage of an anticoccidial drug during early growth, with the expectation that immunity will continue to develop from repeated exposure to wild types of coccidia. This method has never been particularly successful because of the difficulty in controlling all of these factors. Immunity is not necessary in broiler chickens or cage layers. Prevention of infection by anticoccidial drugs is preferred.

Anticoccidial Drugs

Many products are available for prevention or treatment of coccidiosis in chickens and turkeys. Detailed instructions for use are provided by all manufacturers to help users comply with regulatory approvals and management considerations. High dosages may sometimes be used over short periods for treatment or if a high level of exposure is anticipated.

Anticoccidials are given in the feed to prevent disease and the economic loss often associated with subacute infection. Prophylactic use is preferred because most of the damage occurs before signs become apparent, and because drugs cannot completely stop an outbreak. Water medication is generally preferred over feed medication for therapeutic treatment. Antibiotics and increased levels of vitamins A and K are sometimes used in the ration to improve rate of recovery and prevent secondary infections.

Continuous use of anticoccidial drugs promotes the emergence of drug-resistant strains of coccidia. Various programs are used in attempts to slow or stop selection of resistance. For instance, producers may use one anticoccidial continuously through succeeding flocks, rotate anticoccidials every 4-6 mo, or change anticoccidials during a single growout (ie, a shuttle program). While there is little cross-resistance to anticoccidials with different modes of action, there is widespread resistance to most drugs. Change of drug may be beneficial when resistance has been established. "Shuttle programs," in which 1 group of chickens is treated sequentially with different drugs (usually a change between the starter and grower rations), are common practice in many countries, and offer some benefit in reducing emergence of resistance. In the USA, the FDA considers shuttle programs as extra-label usage, but producers may use such programs on the recommendation of a veterinarian.

The effects of anticoccidial drugs may be coccidiostatic, in which growth of intracellular coccidia is arrested but development may continue after drug withdrawal, or coccidiocidal, in which coccidia are killed during their development. Some anticoccidial drugs may be coccidiostatic when given short-term but coccidiocidal when given longterm. Most anticoccidials currently used in poultry production are coccidiocidal.

The natural development of immunity to coccidiosis can be slowed by use of some highly effective anticoccidials. In the production of broilers during a short growout of 37-44 days, this may be of little consequence. However, natural immunity is important in replacement layers because they are likely to be exposed to coccidial infections for extended periods after terminating anticoccidial drugs. Anticoccidial programs for layer and breeder flocks are aimed at allowing immunising infection while guarding against acute outbreaks.

Anticoccidials are commonly withdrawn from broilers 3-7 days before slaughter to meet regulatory requirements and to reduce production costs. Because broilers have varying susceptibility to infection at this point, the risk of coccidiosis outbreaks is increased with longer withdrawal.

Turkeys are given a preventive anticoccidial for confinement-reared birds up to 8-10 wk of age. Older birds are considered less susceptible to outbreaks.

The modes of action of anticoccidial drugs are poorly understood. Some that are better known are described below. Knowledge of mode of action is important in understanding toxicity and side effects.

Amprolium is structurally similar to and is a competitive antagonist of thiamine (vitamin B_1). Because rapidly dividing coccidia have a relatively high requirement for thiamine, amprolium has a safety margin of ~8:1 when used at the highest recommended level in feed. Maximal effect occurs about day 3 of the life cycle of coccidia. Because amprolium has poor activity against some Eimeria spp, its spectrum has been extended by using it in mixtures with the folic acid antagonists, ethopabate and sulfaquinoxaline.

Clopidol and quinolines (eg, decoquinate, methylbenzoquate) halt development of the sporozoites or trophozoites of Eimeria spp by inhibiting the electron transport system within parasite mitochondria. This action is coccidiostatic. Clopidol and quinolines have a broad species spectrum, but resistance may develop rapidly.

Folic acid antagonists include the sulfonamides, 2,4-diaminopyrimidines and ethopabate. These compounds are structural antagonists of folic acid or of para-aminobenzoic acid (PABA), which is a precursor of folic acid. (The host does not synthesize folic acid and has no requirement for PABA.) Coccidia rapidly synthesize nucleic acids, especially during schizogony, which accounts for activity against these stages. Although resistance to antifolate compounds is widespread, they are commonly used for water treatment when clinical signs are already evident. Diaveridine, ormetoprim, and pyrimethamine are active against the protozoan enzyme dihydrofolate reductase. They have synergistic activity with sulfonamides and often are used in mixtures with these compounds.

Halofuginone hydrobromide is related to the antimalarial drug febrifuginone and is effective against asexual stages of most species of Eimeria. It has both coccidiostatic and coccidiocidal effects.

The ionophores (monensin, salinomycin, lasalocid, narasin, maduramicin, and semduramicin) form complexes with various ions, principally sodium, potassium, and calcium, and transport these into and through biological membranes. The ionophores affect both extra-

and intracellular stages of the parasite, especially during the early, asexual stages of parasite development. Drug tolerance was initially slow to emerge, probably because of the biochemically nonspecific way these fermentation products act on the parasite. Recent surveys suggest that drug tolerance is now widespread, but these products remain the most important class of anticoccidials.

Some ionophores depress weight gain when given at or slightly above the recommended levels. Primarily, this is the result of reduced feed consumption, but the reduced growth may be offset by improved feed conversion.

Nicarbazin was the first product to have truly broad-spectrum activity that is still in common use. While not completely understood, the mode of action is thought to be via inhibition of succinate-linked nicotinamide adenine dinucleotide reduction and the energy-dependent transhydrogenase, and the accumulation of calcium in the presence of ATP. Nicarbazin is toxic for layers, and a 4 day withdrawal period is required in broilers. Medicated birds are at increased risk of heat stress in hot weather.

Nitrobenzamides (eg, dinitolmide) exert their greatest coccidiostatic activity against the asexual stages. Efficacy is limited to E tenella and E necatrix unless combined with other products.

Robenidine, a guanidine compound, allows initial intracellular development of coccidia but prevents formation of mature schizonts. It is both coccidiostatic when given short term and coccidiocidal long term. Drug resistance may develop during use. A 5 day withdrawal period is needed to eliminate untoward flavour caused by residues in poultry meat.

Cryptosporidiosis

Cryptosporidiosis is caused by protozoa (phylum Apicomplexa) that are members of the family Cryptosporidiidae and are related to coccidia of the genera Eimeria, Isospora, Sarcocystis, and Toxoplasma. Until recently, it was thought that there were 19 species in the genus Cryptosporidium, but recent research has shown that most are merely species that lack host specificity. Cryptosporidia are parasitic in the intestine of mammals, but in birds they are commonly found in the bursa and in the respiratory tract. Cryptosporidiosis is more severe in turkeys than in chickens and is frequently fatal in quail.

The life cycle of Cryptosporidium is similar to that of other coccidia, involving asexual and sexual phases, and culminates in oocyst production.

In the host, the oocyst forms four sporozoites without sporocysts. The life cycle is not self-limiting (as with other coccidia) because some oocysts are thin-walled and release sporozoites (after trypsin/bile stimulation) that reinfect adjacent tissues. The endogenous cycle is short (4-7 days), the endogenous stages are small (4-7 µm), and the parasites are just beneath the epithelial cell membranes.

In turkeys and chickens, Cryptosporidium have been found in the sinuses, trachea, bronchi, cloaca, and bursa. The respiratory disease causes coughing, gasping, and airsacculitis. Lungs become gray and wet. Signs last several weeks, and death may occur.

Examining tissue scrapings from the bursa, cloaca, and trachea, and finding the characteristic small (5 µm) oocysts can be diagnostic. Concentration of intestinal scrapings using saturated sugar solution and examination by phase-contrast or interference-contrast microscopy is preferred.

There are no satisfactory control measures except isolation and good sanitation. All known anticoccidial drugs are ineffective against Cryptosporidium spp. Unlike Cryptosporidium spp of other mammals, the avian species are not infectious to people.

Coronaviral Enteritis of Turkeys

Etiology and Epidemiology

Coronaviral enteritis is an acute, highly contagious disease of turkeys characterised by sudden onset, marked depression, anorexia, diarrhea, dehydration, and weight loss. Mortality may be high, particularly in poults, but failure to gain body weight in adult birds may be more important economically.

Etiology and Epidemiology

The causative agent is a coronavirus, but the clinical disease is often complicated by other intestinal viral, bacterial, and protozoal infections. Spread is by direct or indirect contact with infected birds or contaminated premises. Droppings of acutely infected birds are rich in virus, and recovered birds may continue to shed lower levels of virus for months. Environmental factors do not appear to influence the occurrence; however, cold temperatures may contribute to the severity of the disease. Cold weather, especially freezing, and high litter moisture increase survival of the virus.

Clinical Findings

A short incubation period, often 48-72 hr, is followed by general depression, anorexia, and diarrhea in the flock. Young poults appear cold, chirp constantly, and seek heat. Feed and water consumption drop markedly, and poults lose weight rapidly. Morbidity and mortality may approach 100% in uncontrolled outbreaks.

Morbidity and mortality are variable in growing and adult turkeys. Profuse diarrhea, with mucoid threads or casts in the droppings, is common. Dehydration and weight loss are often pronounced, and several weeks may be required for normal growth to resume. Cyanosis of the head is common. Breeder hens experience a severe drop in egg production and produce abnormal eggs with chalky shells. Vertical transmission does not occur.

Lesions

Young birds have few lesions other than flaccid, distended intestines that contain excess fluid and gas. Ceca are distended with foamy, pale brown, fetid fluid. Lesions in older birds are more extensive. Skin and musculature are dehydrated, and petechial hemorrhages may be seen on the viscera. Kidneys frequently are swollen and contain an excess of urates, and the pancreas may have multiple, chalky white areas. Severe catarrhal enteritis is common and mucoid casts may be present. The crop may be distended and contain sour-smelling fluid. The spleen is often small and pale gray.

Diagnosis

Although clinical findings and lesions are suggestive, definitive diagnosis requires laboratory techniques including demonstration of coronaviral antigen in intestines of affected birds by direct fluorescent antibody techniques, detection of coronavirus particles in intestinal contents by electron microscopy, reproduction of the disease in naive poults with bacteria-free intestinal filtrates, and negative findings for common bacterial and protozoal infections. Other conditions that may produce similar signs in poults include hexamitiasis (*Hexamitiasis: Introduction*), salmonellosis (*Salmonelloses: Introduction*), inanition, and water deprivation. Other intestinal viruses (which are common in commercial flocks, including rotavirus, reovirus, astrovirus, enterovirus, and possibly others) can cause disease that resembles mild coronaviral enteritis. In older birds, severe larval ascarid infection may cause diagnostic confusion.

Prevention and Treatment

Introduction of virus should be minimised by good management and sanitation practices. Depopulation of problem premises followed by thorough cleaning and disinfection of buildings and equipment is effective in breaking the cycle of infection. Such farms are best cleaned during summer and should be left vacant for e"1 mo.

A commercial vaccine is not available. "Controlled" exposure programs have been used with variable success on some problem farms, but such procedures are not recommended because carrier states may be induced.

The course of disease outbreaks may be altered by good nursing care and judicious use of antibiotics and other drugs to combat secondary bacterial infections and dehydration. Birds in brooder houses should be provided with supplemental heat, and birds on range should be protected from adverse environmental conditions. Antibiotic administration decreases mortality but not the growth suppressant effects. The selection of an antibiotic is empiric at best, but tetracyclines, neomycin, streptomycin, lincomycin, penicillin, and bacitracin are among those used with variable success. Antibiotics may be added to drinking water in combination with calf milk-replacer and electrolyte, eg, 25 lb (11.4 kg) of calf milk-replacer and 450 g of potassium chloride to 100 gal. (380 L) of water. Birds should be medicated for 7-10 days. During and after treatment, birds should be observed closely for secondary crop mycosis, a common sequela of longterm antibiotic therapy.

Chapter 7

Duck Viral Enteritis

Duck Plague

Duck viral enteritis (DVE) is an acute, highly contagious disease of ducks, geese, and swans of all ages, characterised by sudden death, high mortality (particularly among older ducks), and hemorrhages and necrosis in internal organs. It has been reported in domestic and wild waterfowl in Europe, Asia, North America, and Africa, resulting in limited to serious economic losses on domestic duck farms and sporadic, limited to massive die-offs in wild waterfowl.

Etiology, Epidemiology, and Transmission

Field strains of the causative herpesvirus are antigenically similar but vary considerably in pathogenicity. The virus is relatively sensitive to heat and pH; lipid solvents, trypsin, and chymotrypsin inactivate it. It causes intranuclear inclusion bodies in infected tissues and in inoculated cell cultures. In nature, the virus is mainly transmitted from infected to susceptible ducks by direct contact or water and is acquired mainly by the oral route. Parenteral, intranasal, or oral administration of infected tissues can establish experimental infection. Recovered birds may remain carriers, serving as uncontrolled sources of the virus for susceptible ducks.

Clinical Findings

The incubation period is 3-7 days. Sudden high and persistent mortality is often the first sign of the disease. Mortality varies from 5-100% depending on the virulence of the infecting viral strain. Adult ducks usually die in higher proportions than young ones, increasing the economic significance of the disease. Dead males may have prolapse of the penis. Photophobia, inappetence, extreme thirst, droopiness, ataxia, nasal discharge, soiled vents, and watery or bloody diarrhea may be seen. Adult ducks may die in good flesh. In contrast, ducklings frequently show dehydration and weight loss, as well as blue beaks and bloodstained vents. In laying flocks, egg production may drop sharply.

Lesions

Hemorrhages in various tissues and free blood in body cavities indicate severe damage to blood vessels throughout the body. Petechial and ecchymotic hemorrhages on the heart ("paint brush" appearance), liver, pancreas, mesentery, and other organs are characteristic. Specific mucosal eruptions, found in the oral cavity, esophagus, ceca, rectum, and cloaca, undergo progressive alterations during the course of the disease.

Macular hemorrhages initially develop into elevated, yellowish, crusted plaques and organise into green, superficial scabs, which may coalesce into large, patchy, diphtheritic membranes. The mucosal lesions align parallel with the longitudinal folds in the esophagus and with the annular bands in the intestines. All lymphoid organs are affected; necrosis and hemorrhages are apparent. A lesion that can be easily detected on necropsy is a clear, yellow fluid that infiltrates and discolours the subcutaneous tissues from the thoracic inlet to the upper third of the neck. Ruptured yolk and free blood may be found in the abdominal cavity of laying ducks.

Diagnosis

Presumptive diagnosis is based on disease history and lesions. Definitive diagnosis requires laboratory work. Isolation of the virus from liver, spleen, or kidney tissues may be attempted in various cell cultures (preferably primary Muscovy duck embryo fibroblasts or Muscovy duck embryo liver cultures), duck embryos, or ducklings. Inoculating the chorioallantoic membrane of 9 to 14 day old embryonated Muscovy duck eggs may result in isolation of the virus, but this method is not as sensitive as intramuscular inoculation of day-old ducklings. Muscovy ducklings are more susceptible than White Pekin ducklings. Neutralisation with specific antiserum in these systems confirms the identity of the virus. Fluorescent antibody test can demonstrate DVE viral proteins, and PCR, using DVE virus-specific primers, can amplify the viral DNA in duck tissues or inoculated cultured cells. Serologic tests have little value in the diagnosis of acute infections.

Differential diagnoses include duck viral hepatitis, pasteurellosis, necrotic and hemorrhagic enteritis, trauma, drake damage, and various toxicoses. Newcastle disease, avian influenza, and fowlpox may cause similar lesions but are rarely reported in ducks. Established cases should be reported to the appropriate regulatory agency.

Prevention, Treatment, and Control

There is no treatment. Contact with wild, free-flying waterfowl and direct or indirect contact with contaminated birds or material (free-flowing water) should be avoided. Control is effected by depopulation, removal of birds from the infected environment, sanitation, and disinfection.

Prevention is based on maintaining susceptible birds in a disease-free environment or immunisation.

A chicken-embryo-adapted, modified live virus vaccine has been approved for use in domestic ducks, in zoological aviaries, and by private aviculturists.

A 0.5 mL dose is administered subcutaneously or intramuscularly to domestic ducklings >2 wk of age with a booster inoculation a year later. The vaccine is not approved for use in wild ducks. An inactivated vaccine, which appears to be efficacious as the modified live vaccine, has not been tested on a large scale and is not currently licensed.

Hexamitiasis

Hexamitiasis is an acute, catarrhal enteritis of turkeys, pheasants, quail, chukar partridges, and peafowl. The highest mortality occurs in birds 1-9 wk old. Natural infection has not been observed in chickens. Pigeons are susceptible to another species of Hexamita (H columbae). Hexamitiasis is rare in North America.

Etiology

The causative protozoan parasite in turkeys, Hexamita meleagridis, is spindle-shaped, averages 8 × 3 μm, and has 6 anterior and 2 posterior flagella. It has not yet been cultured in experimental media, although it has been grown in the allantoic cavity of developing chicken and turkey embryos. It is transmitted directly by ingestion of contaminated feces. Encysted hexamitids may be more important in transmission than free flagellates. Many survivors become carriers and shed parasites in their droppings.

Clinical Findings and Lesions

The nonspecific signs include watery diarrhea, dry unkempt feathers, listlessness, and rapid weight loss despite the fact that the birds continue to eat. Birds may die in convulsions. Bulbous dilatations of the small intestine (especially duodenum and upper jejunum) filled with watery contents are characteristic. The crypts of Lieberkühn contain myriad H meleagridis, which attach to the epithelial cells by their posterior flagella.

Diagnosis

Diagnosis depends on finding the flagellates by microscopic examination of scrapings of the duodenal and jejunal mucosa. Hexamita spp move with a rapid, darting motion (in contrast to the jerky motion of trichomonads). To avoid contamination of instruments with other cecal protozoa, the duodenum should be opened first. Hexamita spp may be demonstrated in poults that have been dead for several hours if the scrapings are placed in a drop of warm (104°F [40°C]), isotonic saline solution on the slide. Presence of a few Hexamita in birds >10 wk old may be unimportant.

Prevention and Treatment

Because many birds remain carriers, breeder turkeys and poults should be raised on separate premises if possible, preferably with separate attendants. Wire platforms should be used under feeders and waterers. Pheasants and quail may also be carriers.

There is no effective treatment for hexamitiasis, although oxytetracycline (0.22% in the feed for 2 wk) or chlortetracycline (0.022-0.044% in the feed for 2 wk) may be of some benefit.

Necrotic Enteritis

Necrotic enteritis is an acute enterotoxemia. The clinical illness is usually very short and often the only signs are a sudden increase in mortality. The disease primarily affects broiler chickens (2-5 wk old) and turkeys (7-12 wk old) raised on litter but can also affect commercial layer pullets raised in cages.

Etiology and Pathogenesis

The causative agent is the gram-positive, obligate, anaerobic bacteria Clostridium perfringens. It is usually isolated on blood agar, incubated anaerobically at 37°C, on which it produces a double zone of hemolysis. There are 2 primary C perfringens types, A and C, associated with necrotic enteritis in poultry. Toxins produced by the bacteria cause damage to the small intestine, liver lesions, and mortality.

C perfringens is a nearly ubiquitous bacteria readily found in soil, dust, feces, feed, and used poultry litter. It is also a normal inhabitant of the intestines of healthy chickens. The enterotoxemia that results in clinical disease most often occurs either following an alteration in the intestinal microflora or from a condition that results in damage to the intestinal mucosa (eg, coccidiosis, mycotoxicosis, salmonellosis, ascarid larvae). High dietary levels of animal byproducts (eg, fishmeal), wheat, barley, oats, or rye predispose birds to the disease. Anything that promotes excessive bacterial growth and toxin production or slows feed passage rate in the small intestine could promote the occurrence of necrotic enteritis.

Clinical Findings and Lesions

Most often the only sign of necrotic enteritis in a flock is a sudden increase in mortality. However, birds with depression, ruffled feathers, and diarrhea may also be seen. The gross lesions are primarily found in the small intestine (jejunum), which may be ballooned, friable, and contain a foul-smelling, brown fluid. The mucosa is usually covered with a tan to yellow pseudomembrane often referred to as a "Turkish towel" in appearance. This pseudomembrane may extend throughout the small intestine or be only in a localised area. The disease persists in a flock for 5-10 days, and mortality is 2-50%.

Diagnosis

A presumptive diagnosis is based on gross lesions and a gram-stained smear of a mucosal scraping that exhibits large, gram-positive rods. Histologic findings consist of coagulative necrosis of one-third to one-half the thickness of the intestinal mucosa and masses of short, thick bacterial rods in the fibrinonecrotic debris. Isolation of large numbers of C perfringens, from intestinal contents that produce the double zone of hemolysis as described above, can confirm the diagnosis. Double zone hemolysis should not be used as the sole criteria for identification of C perfringens because some strains do not produce both toxins responsible for the hemolysis characteristics. Differential media specifically designed for isolation of C perfringens is available and may be useful for diagnosis.

Necrotic enteritis must be differentiated from lesions produced by Eimeria brunetti and also from ulcerative enteritis. Uncomplicated coccidiosis rarely produces lesions as acute or severe as those seen with necrotic enteritis. Ulcerative enteritis caused by C colinum usually produces focal lesions from the distal portion of the small intestine (ileum) to the ceca and is almost always accompanied by hepatic necrosis.

Prevention, Control, and Treatment

Because C perfringens is nearly ubiquitous, it is important to prevent changes in the intestinal microflora that would promote its growth. This can be accomplished by adding antibiotics in the feed such as virginiamycin (20 g/ton feed), bacitracin (50 g/ton feed), and lincomycin (2 g/ton feed). The addition of anticoccidial compounds, especially of the ionophore class, has been extremely helpful in preventing the coccidial damage that leads to necrotic enteritis. Avoiding drastic changes in feed and minimising the level of fishmeal, wheat, barley, or rye in the diet can also aid in the prevention of necrotic enteritis. Administration of probiotics or competitive exclusion cultures has been used to both prevent and treat clinical necrotic enteritis (presumably by preventing the proliferation of C perfringens). Treatment for necrotic enteritis is most commonly administered in the drinking water, with bacitracin (200-400 mg/gal. for 5-7 days), penicillin (1,500,000 u/gal. for 5 days), and lincomycin (64 mg/gal. for 7 days) most often used. In each case, the medicated drinking water should be the sole source of water. Moribund birds should be removed promptly, as they can serve as a source of toxicosis or infection due to cannibalism.

Rotaviral Infections in Chickens, Turkeys, and Pheasants

Rotaviral infections are characterised by enteritis and diarrhea in young birds, but chickens have been infected without showing clinical signs.

Avian rotaviruses consist of 4 distinct serotypes (A-D). Group A rotaviruses share a common group antigen with mammalian rotaviruses. Group D rotaviruses have been identified only in avian species. The relationships of the other 2 avian serotypes to mammalian serotypes have not been established. Transmission is horizontally by the oral route. Egg transmission has not been reported. Early signs of diarrhea (wet litter), depression, and poor or abnormal appetite can be seen 2-5 days after infection. Dehydration occurs rapidly, and mortality can be as high as 30-50% in pheasants and turkeys. The survivors appear healthy but smaller than normal. Lesions consist of dilated intestines filled with yellowish, watery contents with gas bubbles. Often, the carcass is dehydrated. Mortality is variable and is usually due to dehydration and emaciation.

Early diarrhea and inappetence that sometimes end with death are indicative but not pathognomonic of rotaviral infection. faecal samples or intestinal contents can be examined by electron microscopy with negative staining, either directly or after ultracentrifugation. Numerous rotaviral particles ~70 nm in diametre, with double-shelled capsids, can be seen and are distinguishable from reovirus by their more sharply defined outer edges. For viral isolation in chicken-embryo liver cells or chick kidney cells, faecal material must be treated with trypsin. Isolated rotaviruses belong mostly to serotype A and, in general, do not cause cytopathic effects on primary isolation. The presence of virus can be demonstrated 2-3 days after inoculation by immunofluorescent staining.

No commercial vaccines are available. Thorough cleaning and disinfection of infected houses is advisable to limit infection. There is no specific treatment.

Trichomoniasis

Trichomoniasis in domestic fowl, pigeons, doves, and hawks is characterised, in most cases, by caseous accumulations in the throat and usually by weight loss. It has been termed "canker," "roup," and, in hawks, "frounce."

Etiology

The causative organism is Trichomonas gallinae, a flagellated protozoan that lives in the sinuses, mouth, throat, esophagus, and other organs. It is more prevalent among domestic pigeons and wild doves than among domestic fowl, although severe outbreaks have been reported in chickens and turkeys. Some strains of T gallinae cause high mortality in pigeons and doves. Hawks may become diseased after eating infected birds and commonly show liver lesions, with or without throat involvement. Pigeons and doves transmit the infection to their offspring in contaminated pigeon milk. Contaminated water is probably the most important source of infection for chickens and turkeys.

Clinical Findings

The disease course is rapid. The first lesions appear as small, yellowish areas on the oral mucosa. They grow rapidly and coalesce to form masses that frequently completely block the esophagus and may prevent the bird from closing its mouth. Much fluid may accumulate in the mouth.

There is a watery ocular discharge and, in more advanced stages, exudate about the eyes that may result in blindness. Birds lose weight rapidly, become weak and listless, and sometimes die within 8-10 days. In chronic infections, birds appear healthy, although trichomonads can usually be demonstrated in scrapings from the mucous membranes of the throat.

Lesions

The bird may be riddled with caseous, necrotic foci. The mouth and esophagus contain a mass of necrotic material that may extend into the skull and sometimes through the surrounding tissues of the neck to involve the skin.

In the esophagus and crop, the lesions may be yellow, rounded, raised areas, with a central conical caseous spur, often referred to as "yellow buttons." The crop may be covered by a yellowish, diphtheritic membrane that may extend to the proventriculus.

The gizzard and intestine are not involved. Lesions of internal organs are most frequent in the liver; they vary from a few small, yellow areas of necrosis to almost complete replacement of liver tissue by caseous necrotic debris. Adhesions and involvement of other internal organs appear to be contact extensions of the liver lesions.

Diagnosis

Lesions of T gallinae infection are characteristic but not pathognomonic; those of pox and other infections can be similar. Diagnosis should be confirmed by microscopic examination of a smear of mucus or fluid from the throat to demonstrate the presence of trichomonads.

Trichomonads can be cultured easily in various artificial media such as 0.2% Loeffler's dried blood serum in Ringer's solution or a 2% solution of pigeon serum in isotonic salt solution. Good growth is obtained at 98.6°F (37°C). Antibiotics may be used to reduce bacterial contamination.

Control

Because T gallinae infection in pigeons is so readily transmitted from parent to offspring in the normal feeding process, chronically infected birds should be separated from breeding birds. In pigeons, recovery from infection with a less virulent strain of T gallinae appears to provide some protection against subsequent attack by a more virulent strain. Successful treatments include metronidazole (60 mg/kg body wt) and dimetridazole (50 mg/kg body wt, PO; or in the drinking water at 0.05% for 5-6 days). Neither of these drugs is approved for use in birds in the USA.

Ulcerative Enteritis

Ulcerative enteritis was first diagnosed in bobwhite quail (Colinus virginianus). It also affects chickens, turkeys, pheasants, grouse, and other gallinaceous birds. The disease has also been reported in pigeons. Japanese quail (Coturnix coturnix *japonica)* are resistant, as only experimentally induced cases were reported in highly inbred populations. Marked differences in mortality between males and females suggest that susceptibility is an inheritable trait in *Coturnix* quail. Ulcerative enteritis occurs worldwide and may be acute or chronic.

Etiology

Clostridium colinum is the etiologic agent. It is an anaerobic, fastidious to culture, gram-positive, spore-forming, slightly curved rod, ~1 × 3-4 µm wide, with subterminal, oval spores. In chickens, the disease is a complex that is linked to stress, coccidiosis, infectious bursal disease, and other predisposing factors. To induce experimental disease in quail, >10 viable bacterial cells must be administered PO; chickens inoculated at the same levels are not affected.

Epidemiology

Birds that develop chronic ulcerative enteritis or have recovered from the disease remain carriers. Infection can be introduced by flies feeding on contaminated faecal material or by recovered carrier birds. Infected birds shed the bacterium in their droppings. Bobwhite quail are the most susceptible to this highly contagious disease. Most cases are reported in captive populations of bobwhite quail, suggesting that management plays a role in the incidence of ulcerative enteritis. C colinum spores can survive in the premises for months.

Pathogenesis

After oral infection, the bacterium adheres to the intestinal villi, producing enteritis and ulcers in portions of the small intestine and upper large intestine. Bacilli migrate to the liver via portal circulation, producing necrotic foci that later coalesce into extensive hepatic necrosis.

Infarcts of the spleen are common. Stained smears of the lesions reveal the rod-shaped C colinum microorganism. Although toxigenicity tests in mice have been negative, the role of an in situ-produced toxin in the pathogenesis has been suggested but not demonstrated.

Clinical Findings

In susceptible bobwhite quail, sudden death occurs without signs or weight loss and with up to 100% mortality in just 2-3 days. Acute lesions include hemorrhagic enteritis of the duodenum. In chickens, as well as other game birds, the course of the disease is less severe and is accompanied by anorexia.

Signs are similar to those seen in coccidiosis—depressed, listless birds with humped backs, ruffled feathers, diarrhea, sometimes bloody or watery white droppings, especially in quail in the prolonged course. Chickens recover within 2-3 wk and mortality rarely exceeds 10%.

Lesions

In early disease stages, the most common lesions include small, round ulcers surrounded by hemorrhages in the small intestine, ceca, and upper large intestine. Small ulcers later coalesce to form larger, sometimes perforating ulcers, producing local or diffuse peritonitis. The presence of blood in the gut resembles coccidiosis. Characteristic yellow to gray necrotic foci are the predominant lesions in the hepatic parenchyma. Spleen enlargement with hermorrhages and nectrotic areas may be present.

Diagnosis

Gross postmortem lesions including intestinal ulcerations and yellow to gray necrotising lesions in the liver assist in diagnosis. C colinum can be seen in gram-stained smears of the liver and intestinal lesions. In bacteremic birds, the microorganism can also be found in blood and spleen smears. In chickens, differentiating ulcerative enteritis from coccidiosis (*Coccidiosis: Introduction*) may be difficult as both diseases may be present simultaneously. Necrotic enteritis (*Necrotic*

Enteritis: Introduction) and histomoniasis (*Histomoniasis: Introduction*) may also present a diagnostic problem, but the hepatic lesions of ulcerative enteritis help differentiate it from these diseases. C colinum can be isolated from liver samples cultured in strict anaerobic conditions in prereduced blood glucose-yeast horse plasma medium. A fluorescent antibody test also has been used to accurately diagnose ulcerative enteritis.

Prevention, Treatment, and Control

Bacitracin in the feed at 200 g/ton is used for prevention in quail. Streptomycin (0.006%) and furazolidone (0.02%s) in the feed are effective for treating the disease. Prevention must start with good management practices (eg, avoiding the introduction of new birds into existing flocks. High population density is a predisposing factor. The use of cages is recommended in quail breeding. Sick or dead birds should be removed promptly. Total cleanup between flocks and pest control in and around the premises are good preventive measures.

Avian Campylobacter Infection

Campylobacteriosis is a significant enterocolitis of humans acquired through consumption of undercooked poultry meat contaminated with Campylobacter jejuni.

This organism colonises the intestine of chickens, turkeys, and waterfowl but is generally nonpathogenic in mature poultry. Some strains of C jejuni can cause enteritis and death in newly hatched chicks and poults; however, it has not been possible to satisfy Koch's postulates and reproduce the syndrome previously termed "avian vibrionic hepatitis" by administering isolates of C jejuni to chickens.

Commercial poultry and free-living birds are natural reservoirs of the thermophilic campylobacters (C jejuni, C coli, and C lari) and other poorly defined species. It is estimated that over half of all commercial broiler and turkey flocks harbour C jejuni. The organism has been isolated from numerous birds, including Columbae and domestic and free-living Galliformes and Anseriformes.

C jejuni has been demonstrated in all areas of commercial poultry production. Isolation of the organism is a function of surveillance and ability of laboratory personnel to culture and identify Campylobacter spp.

Etiology and Epidemiology

Campylobacter jejuni is the predominant species associated with foodborne infection derived from poultry. Campylobacter coli and C lari are occasionally recovered from the intestinal tract of poultry and have also been implicated in foodborne infection. Environmental contamination is the source of infection for poults, chicks, and ducklings. Litter can remain infective for long periods, subject to at least a 10% moisture level and neutral pH. Infected chicks and poults become colonised and can continue to excrete C jejuni for their lifetimes. Contaminated water may introduce infection into poultry flocks, and nonchlorinated water derived from a dam, river, or shallow well should be regarded as a possible source. Rats, wild birds, and houseflies can infect flocks; equipment and footwear contaminated with feces from an infected source may also serve as a vehicle of transmission. Once C jejuni has been introduced into the environment, rapid transmission within the flock occurs, with subsequent colonisation of a high proportion of exposed breeders, commercial-meat, or laying-strain poultry. It is unclear whether C jejuni can be transmitted vertically, either on the surface of eggs or by transovarial transmission. It can be isolated from the reproductive tracts of hens and roosters.

Clinical Findings

Many chicks are colonised with Campylobacter spp early in life with no associated clinical signs or pathology. Highly pathogenic isolates derived from people with enterocolitis may induce some mortality in chicks.

Lesions

Gross lesions in challenged chicks include distention of the jejunum, disseminated hemorrhagic enteritis, and in some cases, focal hepatic necrosis. Microscopic lesions include edema of the mucosa of the ileum and cecum with C jejuni in the brush border of enterocytes. Mononuclear infiltration of the submucosa and villous atrophy occur, with intraluminal accumulation of mucus, erythrocytes, and both mononuclear and polymorphonuclear cells. It is unclear whether these findings represent a true clinical syndrome in chicks.

Diagnosis

faecal specimens should be collected using rayon-tipped swabs, then placed in semisolid Cary-Blair transport medium. Enrichment culture of specimens in semisolid motility medium facilitates isolation when small numbers of C jejuni are present in a sample. Campylobacter should be cultured on selective media containing brucella agar base and bovine blood with up to 7 antibiotics that inhibit overgrowth of other Enterobacteriaceae. Thermophilic Campylobacter spp should be cultured at 42°C under microaerophilic conditions for 48 hr. The microaerophilic conditions generally consist of 85% nitrogen, 10% carbon dioxide, and 5% oxygen; however, some strains require a hydrogen-enriched atmosphere (5%). Campylobacter spp of significance in poultry are oxidase- and catalase-positive, indole-negative, and reduce selenite. The thermophilic species may be characterised on the basis of hippurate hydrolysis; nalidixic acid sensitivity is no longer reliable due to the increasing prevalence of fluoroquinolone resistant C jejuni. The Penner or Lior serotyping schemes can be used to classify C jejuni ribotyping, or pulsed-field gel analysis can distinguish among various C jejuni isolates.

Control and Prevention

Because C jejuni does not occur as a specific pathogen under commercial conditions, treatment of poultry flocks is not a consideration. If C jejuni is considered a problem in companion bird aviaries or in exotic species, antibiotics such as erythromycin can be administered in drinking water. Galliformes should receive a dosage of 10-30 mg/kg for 4 consecutive days, and Psittaciformes and exotics should be medicated at 30-40 mg/kg.

Preharvest prevention of Campylobacter infection in commercial species is based on strict biosecurity, decontamination of housing between successive flocks, exclusion of rodents and wild birds, and insect eradication. Chlorination of drinking water to 2 ppm and operation of farms on a strict "all-in/all-out" basis occasionally reduces the prevalence of infection. In the context of commercial production in the USA where earth-floored housing is used and litter is recycled, preharvest control of C jejuni is impractical. Innovative methods of prevention, such as competitive inhibition or the use of vaccines, are under intensive investigation, but are unlikely to be available for commercial application in the near future. Withholding feed from broilers and turkeys for at least 12 hr before slaughter and thorough decontamination of transport coops and modules reduce faecal contamination and lower the level of C jejuni introduced into processing plants.

Zoonotic Risk

C jejuni is a major source of foodborne enteritis in consumers; contaminated, undercooked poultry is responsible for >50% of cases investigated. The condition was recognised in the mid 1970s, and the significance of the organism has become apparent with improved methods of isolation and identification. Nonchlorinated ground water, unpasteurised milk, young diarrheic pets, and contaminated beef and pork products may also be responsible for infection of people.

Improved washing of carcasses, use of counter-flow scalding, elimination of immersion chillers, and reduction in manual handling by installation of advanced automated equipment can reduce C jejuni contamination. Chemical disinfectants, such as glutaraldehyde (0.125%) and succinic acid (3%), and organic compounds, such as lactic and acetic acids, may be used to destroy C jejuni.

Gamma irradiation at levels of 1-3 kGy effectively eliminates C jejuni from poultry carcasses and products. Irradiation using cobalt 60 and electron beam generation are cost-effective procedures, which are endorsed by a joint United Nations Committee of the Food and Agricultural Organisation, the International Atomic Energy Agency, and the World Health Organisation. However, irradiation is not well accepted by American consumers. Currently, the only measure to reduce the risk of C jejuni infection to consumers is thorough cooking of poultry to achieve a core temperature of 74°C for 1 min. This ensures destruction of C jejuni. Concurrent hygienic storage, handling, and preparation are necessary to prevent contamination of prepared foods, work surfaces, and utensils by raw poultry and other meats.

Avian Chlamydiosis

Psittacosis, Ornithosis, Parrot Fever

Avian chlamydiosis can be an inapparent subclinical infection or acute, subacute, or chronic disease of wild and domestic birds characterised by respiratory, digestive, or systemic infection. Infections occur worldwide and have been identified in at least 150 avian species, particularly colonial nesting birds (eg, egrets, herons), ratites, caged birds (primarily psittacines), raptors, and poultry. Among poultry, turkeys, ducks, and pigeons are most often affected; infection of chickens is infrequent. The disease is a significant cause of economic loss and human exposure in European duck flocks. Longterm inapparent infections lasting for months to years are common and considered the normal chlamydia-host relationship; 10-30% of surveyed avian populations may be found positive. The same strain may cause mild disease or asymptomatic infection in one species, but severe or fatal disease in another species.

Avian chlamydiosis is a zoonotic disease that can affect people following exposure to air- or dustborne organisms when infected birds are in flocks or processed, or when organisms are shed from the digestive or respiratory tracts of infected birds confined in breeding aviaries, lofts, or wholesale or retail outlets.

Human disease most often results from exposure to psittacines or pigeons and can occur even if there is only brief proximity to a single infected bird. When workers are exposed to infected turkeys or ducks at processing, increased absenteeism due to acute respiratory disease often occurs ~1 wk after a flock with a high condemnation rate due to airsacculitis has been processed. Some individuals, especially pregnant women and those with impaired immunity, are more susceptible than others. The illness in people is usually respiratory and characterised by abrupt onset of flu-like symptoms; pneumonia, organ failure, and death can result if the disease is severe or left untreated. Precautions should be taken when examining a dead infected bird (eg, detergent disinfectant to wet feathers, fan-exhausted examining hood, dust mask or plastic face shield, and gloves) to avoid exposure.

Etiology and Epidemiology

A recent taxonomic revision resulted in the causative organism being renamed Chlamydophila psittaci (formerly Chlamydia psittaci). The name of the disease resulting from infection with C psittaci remains avian chlamydiosis. C psittaci is an obligate intracellular bacterium. All strains of chlamydia share an identical genus-specific antigen in their lipopolysaccharide but often differ in the composition of other cell-wall antigens, providing a basis for serotypic identification. Currently, 8 serotypes are recognised; 6 (A-F) infect avian species and are distinct from mammalian chlamydia serotypes. Each avian serotype tends to be associated with certain types of birds. Serotype D is highly virulent for turkeys and can cause mortality of 30% or higher. Serotypes B and E are most frequently recovered from wild birds. Avian serotypes are capable of infecting people and other mammals.

Respiratory discharges or feces from infected birds contain elementary bodies that are resistant to drying and can remain infective for several months. Airborne particles and dust spread the organism. After inhalation or ingestion, elementary bodies attach to microvilli on mucosal epithelial cells and are internalised by endocytosis. Elementary bodies within endosomes in the cell cytoplasm differentiate into metabolically active, noninfectious reticulate bodies that divide and multiply, eventually forming numerous infectious, metabolically inactive elementary bodies. Newly formed elementary bodies are released from the host cell by lysis.

Possible sources of C psittaci include infected birds, asymptomatic carriers, vertical transmission from infected hens, infected rodents, and contaminated feed. Stressors and concurrent infections, especially those causing immunosuppression, can initiate shedding in latently infected birds and may cause recurrence of clinical disease. Carriers often shed the organism intermittently for extended periods. Persistence of C psittaci in the nasal glands of chronically infected birds may be an important source of organisms. Transmission is faecal-oral or by inhalation. The incubation period typically is 3-10 days but may be up to 2 mo in older birds or following low exposure.

Host and microbial factors, route and intensity of exposure, and treatment determine clinical course.

Clinical Findings and Lesions

Severity of clinical signs and lesions depends on the virulence of the organism and susceptibilty of the bird; asymptomatic infections are common. Nasal and ocular discharges, conjunctivitis, sinusitis, green to yellow-green droppings, fever, inactivity, ruffled feathers, weakness, inappetence, and weight loss can be seen in clinically affected birds. Necropsy findings in acute infections include serofibrinous polyserositis (airsacculitis, pericarditis, perihepatitis, peritonitis), pneumonia, hepatomegaly, and splenomegaly. Multiple pale foci and/or petechial hemorrhages can be seen in the liver and spleen. Similar lesions are seen in other systemic bacterial infections and are not specific for avian chlamydiosis. Multifocal necrosis in the liver and spleen is associated with large, granular, basophilic intracytoplasmic inclusions, occasional heterophils, and increased mononuclear cells (macrophages, lymphocytes, plasma cells) in hepatic sinusoids and splenic sinuses. Necrosis results from direct cell lysis or vascular damage. The latter is also the source of the generalised serofibrinous exudation. Enlargement and discoloration of the spleen or liver characterise chronic infections. Necrosis and inclusions are not seen, but the mononuclear cell response is present in these birds. Lesions are usually absent in latently infected birds, even though C psittaci is often being shed.

Diagnosis

Because of the variety of clinical presentations and common occurrence of latently infected carriers, no single diagnostic test can reliably determine infection. Procedures to detect the organism or antibodies are used. In general, the more acute the disease, the greater the number of infective organisms and the easier it is to make a diagnosis. When birds are acutely ill, clinical findings, including hematology, clinical chemistries, and radiology or typical gross lesions, are adequate for a tentative diagnosis. The organism can often be identified in impression smears of affected tissues stained by Giemsa, Gimenez, or Macchiavello's methods.

Antigen detection methods include immunohistochemistry (immunofluorescence, immunoperoxidase), ELISA, and PCR. Immunohistochemistry is accurate when done by a skilled person and the number of organisms is sufficient for detection. ELISA kits are available commercially and are relatively inexpensive, easy to use, and have good specificity, but low sensitivity. They are most useful when birds are clinically ill. PCR tests have been developed but are not widely available and require further evaluation. Multiple samples collected for 3-5 days are recommended for detection of intermittent shedding by asymptomatic birds.

Confirmation requires isolation and identification of C psittaci in chick embryos or cell cultures (BGM, L929, Vero) at a qualified laboratory. Cloacal, choanal, oropharyngeal, conjunctival, or faecal swabs from live birds or tissues (eg, liver, spleen, serosal membranes) from dead birds should be submitted. Sampling from mutiple sites and over several days will increase detection of intermittent shedding. Freezing, drying, improper handling, and certain transport media can affect viability. Refrigeration; placing specimens in sealed plastic bags or other containers; using a special buffer prepared from sucrose, phosphate, and glutamase (SPG buffer); and prompt delivery of fresh specimens are preferred. The laboratory should be contacted for directions on submitting samples before they are sent. Concurrent infections with other more easily diagnosed diseases (eg, colibacillosis, pasteurellosis, herpesvirus infections, mycotic diseases, etc.) may mask chlamydial infection. Laboratory and clinical findings should be correlated with each other. Chlamydiosis must be distinguished from other respiratory and systemic diseases of birds.

Antibodies may or may not be detectable depending on the test used, degree and stage of infection, and treatment of the bird. Interpretation of titres from single serum samples is difficult. A 4-fold increase in titres between paired acute and convalescent samples is diagnostic, and high titres in a majority of samples from several birds in a population are sufficient for a presumptive diagnosis. Serologic methods include direct and modified direct complement fixation, latex agglutination, elementary body agglutination, and direct and competitive ELISA. ELISA provides the greatest sensitivity and specificity compared with culture. The elementary body agglutination test detects IgM and is useful for determining recent infection.

Prevention and Treatment

Local governmental regulations should be followed wherever applicable. No effective vaccine for use in birds is available. Treatment will prevent mortality and shedding but cannot be relied on to eliminate latent infection; shedding may recur. Tetracyclines (chlortetracycline, oxytetracycline, doxycycline) are the antibiotics of choice. Drug resistance to tetracyclines is rare, but reduced sensitivity requiring higher dosages is becoming more common. Tetracyclines are bacteriostatic and only effective against actively multiplying organisms, making extended treatment times (from 2-6 wk, during which minimum-inhibitory concentrations in blood are consistently maintained) necessary.

Outbreaks in poultry flocks are not common. Treating infected flocks with chlortetracycline at 400-750 g/ton for a minimum of 2 wk before processing has effectively eliminated potential risk of infection for plant employees.

In companion birds, use of chlortetracycline-medicated feeds for 45 days is a standard recommendation for imported birds. Difficulties in palatability of the feed itself or high level of antibiotic necessary for adequate blood levels have limited its use. Long-acting oxytetracycline at 50-100 mg/kg, IM, every 2-3 days for 30 days, provides adequate continuous blood levels and results in elimination of shedding within 24 hr. However, muscle necrosis at injection sites may be extensive, which limits the usefulness of this treatment. Doxycycline in a formulation for IM use has been given at 75-100 mg/kg as a series of 7 injections over a 6 wk period. Addition of doxycycline to feeds can also result in adequate blood levels and has less effect on normal intestinal flora than does chlortetracycline. Supportive care for acutely affected birds also aids recovery.

Appropriate biosecurity practices are necessary for controlling the introduction and spread of chlamydiae in an avian population. Minimal standards include quarantine and examination of all new birds, traffic control to minimise cross-contamination, isolation and treatment of affected and contact birds, thorough cleaning and disinfection of premises and equiment (preferably with small units managed on an all-in/all-out basis), provision of uncontaminated feed, maintenance of records on all bird movements, and continual monitoring for presence of chlamydial infection.

The organism is susceptible to heat and most disinfectants (eg, 1:1,000 quaternary ammonium chloride, 1:100 bleach solution, 70% alcohol, etc.), but is resistant to acid and alkali. A voluntary cooperative improvement plan leading to certification of companion birds derived from chlamydia-free breeders has been developed.

Avian Nephritis Viral Infections

Avian nephritis viral infections are contagious infections of chickens and turkeys characterised by renal damage and visceral urate deposits, growth retardation, runting-stunting syndrome, and limited mortality (2-6%). They are seen mainly in chickens <7 days old, but interstitial nephritis can be observed in chicks up to 4 wk old. These infections have been reported worldwide. Subclinical infections are common and have been detected by serologic surveys in some SPF flocks.

Etiology and Transmission

The causal viruses are avian nephritis virus (ANV, an astrovirus), ANV-like viruses, and related enterovirus-like viruses (ELV). Strains vary in virulence and in antigenicity. Transmission occurs by direct or indirect contact. Indirect evidence suggests that egg transmission may occur. Infection can be transmitted by oral administration of virus to day-old birds. Virus is consistently isolated from the kidneys or the feces during the first 10 days after infection.

Nephropathogenic strains of infectious bronchitis virus (*Infectious Bronchitis: Introduction*) also cause interstitial nephritis. Therefore, when nephritis is diagnosed, it is necessary to isolate the causative agent.

Clinical Findings

Clinical signs vary from none to the so-called runting-stunting syndrome. Diarrhea and growth retardation are common in broilers. Outbreaks with mortality of 2-6% can occur in chicks newly hatched up to 7 days old; cardinal necropsy findings are renal damage and visceral urate deposits (baby chick nephropathy).

Lesions

Nephritis is a common necropsy finding. Gross and microscopic lesions are often seen in the kidneys. Swelling, paleness, or yellowish discoloration with excessive urate deposition is frequent. Histologic lesions consist of a degeneration of the epithelial cells with infiltration of granulocytes, interstitial lymphocyte infiltration, and moderate fibrosis. In the latter stages, lymphoid follicles develop.

Some ELV induce only intestinal lesions varying from decreased length of the microvillus border to total desquamation of the intestinal epithelium.

Diagnosis

ANV and related viruses may be isolated by inoculation of suspected material (kidney or rectal contents) in the yolk sac of SPF chick embryos and in chick kidney cells. However, many ANV, ANV-like, and ELV viruses are difficult to isolate. The best method of detection is by electron microscopic examination of faecal preparations. Direct immunofluorescence performed on kidney sections is also a useful diagnostic procedure and allows quick differentiation from infectious bronchitis virus. Serologic diagnosis can be made using indirect immunofluorescence, seroneutralisation, or ELISA tests.

Treatment and Prevention

There is no effective treatment. General hygienic precautions are the only applicable preventive measures.

Chapter 8

Avian Spirochetosis

Avian Borreliosis

Avian spirochetosis is an acute, febrile, septicemic, bacterial disease that affects a wide variety of birds.

Etiology, Epidemiology, and Transmission

The causal organism, Borrelia anserina, is an actively motile spirochete, ~0.2-0.3 μm × 8-20 μm, and consists of 5-8 loosely arranged coils. Cultivation in vitro is difficult. Borrelia will grow on Barbour-Stoenner-Kelly medium, but loses virulence after 12 passages. It can also be propagated in embryonating duck or chick embryos or in young ducks or chicks.

Spirochetosis is found in temperate or tropical regions, wherever the biologic vectors are found. The most common vector is Argas (Persicargas) persicus, the "cosmopolitan" fowl tick, but other Argas spp transmit the disease in different geographic areas. In the western USA, a highly efficient vector is A sanchezi.

Diverse immunologic and serologic types of B anserina have been demonstrated in many areas. Recovery from one type confers solid immunity against the homologous types for e"1 yr, but not against heterologous strains. Relapses, such as occur with some human Borrelia infections, are unknown in B anserina infection of birds; any reinfection can be attributed to a heterologous type.

Generally, an infected Argas tick can transmit the disease at every feeding and maintains the infection throughout larval, nymphal, and adult stages. The ticks also transmit the infection transovarially, ie, the F_1 larvae are infective. Ticks remain infected despite feeding on chicks hyperimmune to B anserina or on chicks with high blood levels of chemotherapeutic agents effective against Borrelia. Other vectors (lice, mosquitos, some species of ticks, inanimate objects) can transmit the spirochete mechanically to a susceptible host whenever the piercing apparatus becomes contaminated with blood that contains Borrelia. Ingestion of bile-stained faecal droppings containing the spirochete, contamination of feed or water, and cannibalism during spirochetemia can result in infection. After the bite of an infected tick, the incubation period is ~3-12 days.

Clinical Findings

Marked enlargement and mottling of the spleen is the most characteristic lesion. Signs are highly variable, depending on the virulence of the spirochete, and may be absent. Signs include listlessness, depression, somnolence, moderate to marked shivering, and increased thirst. Young birds are affected more severely than older ones. During the initial stages of the disease, there is usually a green or yellow diarrhea with increased urates. The course of the disease is 1-2 wk. Mild strains are common. However, in many tick-infested geographic areas, morbidity can approach 100% and mortality may be 33-77%. Egg production in layers or breeders may be reduced by 5-10%, with a higher number of small eggs.

Lesions

An enlarged spleen with petechial or ecchymotic hemorrhages, not unlike spleens in marble spleen disease of pheasants (*Hemorrhagic Enteritis of Turkeys and Marble Spleen Disease of Pheasants: Introduction*), is present. However, a contrasting situation may be seen in Mongolian pheasants, in which the spleen is reported to be small and pale. Occasionally, the liver may be swollen and contain focal areas of necrosis. Kidneys may be enlarged and pale. A green, catarrhal enteritis is common.

Diagnosis

Diagnosis depends on demonstration of Borrelia in the blood, either as actively motile during darkfield microscopy, or as stained spirochetes in Giemsa-stained blood smears. In young birds, the Borrelia may reach vast numbers per oil-immersion field and persist for several days. Older birds usually have low numbers of Borrelia that are detected only with difficulty, or not at all, and that persist for only 1-2 days. Anaemia is common and results in increased numbers of immature RBC.

Agar-gel diffusion and various serologic tests have been described but are of questionable value due to diverse serotypes that exist in some localities. Specific agglutinins clump the spirochetes in successively larger clumps during the terminal stages of the disease. Agglutination-lysis then begins to disintegrate these clumps, and spirochetal degradation products are liberated, which may result in pyrexia. Death occurs most often 1-3 days after Borrelia disappear from the bloodstream. Spirochetal antibodies are readily detected in yolks of eggs laid by infected hens.

Treatment and Control

Several antibacterial agents are effective. The most widely used are penicillin derivatives, but the streptomycins, tetracyclines, and tylosin are also effective. The antibiotics can be completely efficacious if begun when the number of spirochetes per oil-immersion field is low or moderate; however, if large numbers of spirochetes are present in the bloodstream, the sudden liberation of large quantities of spirochetal degradation products can result in higher mortality than no treatment.

Control must be directed against the biologic vector. Argas ticks are notable for their long lifespan, ability to survive for extended periods without a blood meal, efficiency in transmitting the spirochete, and ability to remain securely hidden in cracks and crevices often beyond the effective reach of pesticides. Accordingly, control is difficult. A combination of tick eradication and immunisation is the most effective means of control.

Immunisation can be highly successful and, next to eradication of the biologic vector, is the preferred method of control. Bacterins prepared from local strains of Borrelia have been used with success. Vaccines may be prepared from formalin- or phenol-inactivated material from lysates of blood, tissues, embryos, or eggs infected with B anserina, and may be lyophilised or liquid. Whole-egg propagated bacterins are usually given in 1 or 2 IM injections. Little if any cross-protection is afforded to different serotypes. Birds normally have protective immunity after recovering from natural infection.

Listeriosis

Listeriosis is quite rare in birds and usually occurs as a septicemia or sometimes as a localised encephalitis. Encephalitis combined with septicemia has been seen in young geese. Chickens, turkeys, geese, ducks, canaries, and parrots appear to be the most commonly affected avian species.

In workers at poultry-processing plants, conjunctivitis due to Listeria monocytogenes has been linked to handling of apparently normal but infected chickens. Human infections have also resulted from consumption of contaminated poultry or poultry products. Abortions and congenitally infected babies have been associated with handling of L monocytogenes -positive birds or those that have died with the disease, but these cases were not confirmed.

Etiology and Epidemiology

L monocytogenes is a gram-positive, coccoid to bacillus-shaped, nonsporeforming bacteria that tends to form long filaments, particularly in older cultures. Based on somatic and flagellar antigens, several serotypes have been described. L monocytogenes can be cultured on blood and tryptose agar or brain-heart infusion. It is widely distributed among avian species. The organism is common in feces and soil, with numbers increasing in late winter and early spring. It has been isolated from apparently normal birds and from birds dying of causes other than uncomplicated listeriosis; therefore, it is possible that carrier birds play an important role in the perpetuation of the disease in birds and mammals. It is commonly associated with concurrent diseases such as coccidiosis, infectious coryza, salmonellosis, and parasitic infections demonstrating the largely opportunistic character of the organism.

Clinical Findings

Young birds appear to be more susceptible than mature ones. Transmission and subsequent infections occur by ingestion of contaminated nasal secretions, feces, and soil. Infection can also occur via inhalation and wound contamination. In most avian species, the incubation period has not been documented; in turkeys, it is 16 hr to 52 days. Frequently, L monocytogenes infections are subclinical. Chickens and turkeys are relatively resistant to natural infection. However, signs of infection are suggestive of a septicemia and include depression, listlessness, and peracute death. In this form, it is common to find only dead birds. In the subacute and chronic forms, signs are related to encephalitis and include torticollis, stupor, paresis, and paralysis. Adult birds may die suddenly with septicemia, while young birds tend to have chronic infections. Emaciation and diarrhea are seen in some affected birds.

Lesions

In uncomplicated listeriosis, lesions include multiple areas of degeneration and necrosis of the myocardium with congestion, increased pericardial fluid, and pericarditis. Petechial hemorrhages can be seen in the proventriculus and heart. Splenomegaly and hepatomegaly with bile retention and focal areas of necrosis are common. In the encephalitic form, no gross brain lesions are seen; microscopically, however, gliosis in the cerebellum with microabscesses containing gram-positive bacteria are present in the midbrain and medulla.

Diagnosis

Listeriosis can be suspected based on the history, clinical signs, necropsy lesions, and microscopic observation of the bacteria in the myocardial fibrils, hepatocytes, or both.

The diagnosis can be confirmed by isolation from the blood, liver, heart, spleen, or brain of a gram-positive, nonacid-fast, nonsporeforming bacillus that is catalase-positive, motile, aerobic, and that ferments sugars.

Isolation by direct culture of the affected tissues may not be successful because of low concentration of organisms in the tissues; however, recovery increases significantly if a portion of the specimen is refrigerated for 4-8 wk and subcultured weekly. Chick embryos are readily infected and can be used for organism identification.

Differential diagnoses include colibacillosis, pasteurellosis, erysipelas, velogenic viscerotropic Newcastle disease, and many other acute and chronic bacterial diseases.

Treatment and Control

The organism is often resistant to many of the commonly used antibiotics. However, the tetracyclines have been efficacious in both the acute and subacute forms when given at 25 mg/kg, PO, sid for 1 wk. Treatment of the chronic form is usually unsuccessful. Widespread use of antimicrobials in the feed for growth promotion may have prophylactic value. Rigid sanitation and disinfection procedures with culling and isolation of affected birds may be helpful. Prevention should focus on identifying and eliminating the source of infection.

Malabsorption Syndrome

Runting-stunting Syndrome, Pale Bird Syndrome

Malabsorption syndrome is characterised by stunted growth and a lack of skin pigmentation in growing chickens, most commonly meat type or broilers. It has been identified in virtually all countries in which intensive poultry production occurs.

Etiology and Transmission

Mycotoxins and several viruses, including enteroviruses, parvoviruses, astroviruses, caliciviruses, arenaviruses, and reoviruses have been implicated. Although the etiology is believed to be complex, only mycotoxins, enteroviruses, and reoviruses have thus far been identified as potential etiologic factors.

The specific feedborne mycotoxins involved and concentration needed to induce the syndrome are not well understood. Numerous enteric viruses are prevalent worldwide in commercially produced poultry. Transmission of viruses occurs via faecal-oral routes.

Clinical Findings

The disease is typically recognised in broiler chicks 1-3 wk old. It is characterised by stunted growth; lack of pigmentation in the skin, feet, or beak; slow feathering; broken or twisted feathers; undigested feed in the feces; and/or poor feed conversion ratios.

Diarrhea is common during the initial phases. Severely affected birds do not respond immediately to changes in feed or management practices and are usually culled from flocks before processing.

Lesions

The severity and type of lesions resulting from both field and laboratory infections vary with the particular agents or combinations of agents involved. Lesions often include enlarged proventriculi, small gizzards, and orange mucus in the small-intestinal lumen. No consistent microscopic lesions are found. Encephalomalacia or rickets may be seen occasionally, presumably as a result of malabsorption or malassimilation of nutrients.

Diagnosis

Clinical signs and lesions permit a presumptive diagnosis, although a similar gross appearance can be caused by a retrovirus. More conclusive diagnostic evidence includes finding either viruses in the lesions or dietary toxins.

Prevention and Control

There is no effective treatment for severely affected birds. Sanitation and disinfection will reduce the burden of challenge caused by multiple infectious organisms. There are no vaccines that will prevent malabsorption syndrome. Reovirus vaccines can prevent the stunting and poor feed conversions that occur with pathogenic reovirus infections. Feeds should be analysed for dietary toxins, and high levels of toxins should not knowingly be fed to commercial poultry.

Mycoplasmosis

Several Mycoplasma spp have been isolated from avian hosts; M gallisepticum, M iowae, M meleagridis, and M synoviae are the most important. Mycoplasmas are fastidious bacteria, 0.3-0.8 μm in diametre; they lack a cell wall and require a rich growth medium containing serum. They do not survive for more than a few days outside the host and are vulnerable to common disinfectants. Each has distinctive epidemiologic and pathologic characteristics.

Mycoplasma Gallisepticum Infection

M gallisepticum infection is commonly designated as chronic respiratory disease in chickens and as infectious sinusitis in turkeys. Infection may also be seen in pheasants, chukar partridges, and peafowl. Infection in pigeons, quail, ducks, geese, and psittacine birds should be considered. Passerine-type birds are quite resistant, although M gallisepticum is the major cause of natural outbreaks of conjunctivitis in wild house finches (Carpodacus mexicanus) in the eastern USA. The disease is worldwide. Its effects are most severe in large commercial operations during winter.

M gallisepticum is the most pathogenic avian mycoplasma; however, strains may differ markedly in virulence. Primary isolation is made in enriched broth medium containing 10-15% serum, then plated on agar. Typical colonies are identified by immunofluorescence.

Transmission, Epidemiology, and Pathogenesis

In the USA, most breeder flocks are free of M gallisepticum, and outbreaks are due to lateral transmission from infected chickens; however, in some parts of the world, egg transmission is a major source of infection. The incidence of egg transmission is highly variable, ranging up to 30-40% during the first 2 mo after infection of susceptible birds in production. The transmission rate then lessens and is inconsistent (0-5%) until the end of production. Birds infected before the onset of production transmit through the egg at a much lower rate, if at all.

The infection may be dormant in the infected chick for days to months, but when the flock is stressed, aerosol transmission occurs rapidly and infection spreads through the flock. Live virus vaccination, natural virus infection, cold weather, or crowding may initiate the spread. In addition, the infection may be carried by personnel (especially from an infected to a clean flock), fomites, or introduction of infected birds. In many flocks, the source of infection cannot be determined.

The epithelium of the upper air passages is most susceptible to infection; however, in severe, acute disease the infection is also found in the lower respiratory tract. There is a marked interaction between respiratory viruses, Escherichia coli, and M gallisepticum in the pathogenesis of chronic respiratory disease. Once infected, birds remain carriers for life.

Clinical Findings

In chickens, infection may be inapparent or result in varying degrees of respiratory distress, with slight to marked rales, difficulty breathing, coughing, and/or sneezing. Morbidity is high and mortality low in uncomplicated cases. Nasal discharge and frothiness about the eyes may be present. In turkeys, the disease is generally more severe than in chickens, and swelling of the paranasal sinus is common. Feed efficiency and weight gains are reduced. Broilers and market turkeys may suffer high condemnations at processing due to airsacculitis. In laying flocks, birds may fail to reach peak egg production, and the overall production rate is lower than normal.

Lesions

Uncomplicated M gallisepticum infections in chickens result in relatively mild sinusitis, tracheitis, and airsacculitis. E coli infections are often concurrent and result in severe air sac thickening and turbidity, with exudative accumulations, fibrinopurulent pericarditis, and perihepatitis, particularly in broilers. Turkeys develop severe mucopurulent sinusitis and varying degrees of tracheitis and airsacculitis. The mucous membranes are thickened, hyperplastic, necrotic, and infiltrated with inflammatory cells. Lymphofollicular areas are found in the submucosa.

Diagnosis

Agglutination reactions and ELISA are commonly used for diagnosis. M gallisepticum should be confirmed by isolation and identification, PCR, or hemagglutination-inhibition because nonspecific false agglutination reactions are common, especially after the inoculation of inactivated, oil-emulsion vaccines or M synoviae infection. Isolates must be identified, because birds may also be infected with nonpathogenic Mycoplasma spp. PCR is commonly used to rapidly detect the organism in upper respiratory tissues. Newcastle disease, infectious bronchitis, influenza, and other respiratory pathogens should be considered in the differential diagnosis.

Treatment and Control

In the field, many cases of M gallisepticum infection are complicated by other pathogenic bacteria; thus, effective treatment must also attack the secondary invader. Most strains of M gallisepticum are sensitive to a number of antibiotics, such as chlortetracycline, erythromycin, oxytetracycline, spectinomycin, tiamulin, tylosin, or a fluoroquinolone such as enrofloxacin. Antibiotic is usually given in the feed or water for 5-7 days; however, in turkeys, antibiotic may be given initially by injection, followed by feed or water medication. Antibiotics may alleviate the clinical signs and lesions but do not eliminate infection.

Eradication of M gallisepticum from chicken and turkey breeding stock is well advanced in the USA and several other countries. The most effective control program is to identify breeders without serum agglutination or ELISA titres and to maintain seronegative stock. In valuable breeding stock, treatment of eggs, usually with tylosin or heat, may be used to eliminate egg transmission to progeny. Medication is not a good long- term control method but is of value in treating individual infected flocks.

The use of birds free of M gallisepticum is desirable, but infection in multiple-age commercial egg farms where depopulation is not feasible is a problem. An inactivated, oil-emulsion bacterin is available in most countries; it prevents egg production losses but not infection. A live vaccine has been licensed in the USA for use in infected, multiple-age layer flocks but may be used only with permission of the state veterinarian. The vaccine consists of a mild strain of M gallisepticum (F-strain) and is usually given at ~10-14 wk of age. F-strain is of low pathogenicity for chickens but is fully virulent for turkeys. Vaccinated birds remain carriers, and immunity lasts through the laying season. Recently, 2 nonpathogenic live vaccine strains (6/85 and ts-11) have been introduced; these strains offer the advantage of improved safety and are in widespread use in commercial layers.

Mycoplasma Iowae Infection

M iowae was originally thought to be of low pathogenicity in producing air sac lesions in chickens and turkeys, but it is a potentially important cause of reduced hatchability in turkeys. Antigenicity and pathogenicity vary considerably among M iowae strains. M iowae is resistant to 1% bile salts, and an enriched medium similar to those used for other avian mycoplasmas is suitable.

Infection was common in turkey flocks in Europe and North America, but the infection rate has now been reduced by intensive eradication efforts in breeding stocks. It is a relatively uncommon infection of chickens. M iowae is egg transmitted, but little is known of other aspects of its epidemiology.

Many strains of M iowae are lethal to turkey embryos. After experimental inoculation of young poults, stunting, poor feathering, and various skeletal deformities such as tenosynovitis and chondrodystrophy develop, but the mechanism is unknown. These effects have not been recognised in the field, probably because most infected birds die before hatching. Older birds appear to be quite resistant.

Clinical Findings, Lesions, and Diagnosis

Affected turkey breeder flocks show no clinical signs other than reduced hatchability (usually 2-5%). In many flocks, the hatchability returns to normal after 1-2 mo.

Most embryos die during the mid to late stages of incubation. Dead turkey embryos are edematous, congested, and stunted; they may have clubbed down. Poults challenged in ovo or at 1 day of age may develop various skeletal deformities such as rotated tibia, deviated toes, chondrodystrophy, or erosion of the articular cartilage of the hock joint. Feathers may also be poorly developed. Chicks challenged at 1 day of age may develop tenosynovitis and ruptured tendons.

Turkeys apparently have a poor antibody response, and no reliable serologic test is available. Diagnosis relies on isolation and identification of the causative agent.

Treatment and Control

The best method of control is to maintain flocks free of M iowae; however, because serology is unreliable, this may be difficult. Dipping hatching eggs in solutions of enrofloxacin has significantly reduced losses in hatchability.

Mycoplasma Meleagridis Infection

M meleagridis infection is a widespread, egg-transmitted disease of turkeys found worldwide. The primary lesion in the progeny is airsacculitis. M meleagridis is thought to be a specific pathogen for turkeys, and the organism is commonly found in the respiratory and reproductive tracts. It has been eradicated in most basic breeder and many commercial flocks.

M meleagridis was recognised as a pathogen of turkeys after widespread elimination of the bacteria from breeding stock.

Transmission and Pathogenesis

Infection is established primarily through egg transmission, which can be as high as 30-50% or higher early in the production cycle. However, transmission of M meleagridis is also related to genital contact. Early infections usually become quiescent at sexual maturity. In the tom, the phallus and adjacent tissues are infected and contaminate semen, thus infecting the vagina of the hen. Hens may retain infection in the bursa of Fabricius, which serves as a source of infection of the reproductive tract after rupture of the cloacal-vaginal occluding membrane at puberty. Infection ascends the reproductive system and may reach the surface of the ovary. The high rate of egg transmission of M meleagridis is from infection of the reproductive tract being incorporated into the egg after ovulation. Infection of the respiratory tract leads to transmission among birds in young flocks and may be a factor in the spread to flocks previously free of infection. Hatchery transmission is also possible.

The marked difference in the pathogenicity of various strains of M meleagridis results in variable clinical manifestations. The high incidence of air sac infection in poults suggests a symbiotic host-parasite relationship. M meleagridis may be involved in crooked necks and leg deformities, but the pathogenesis of this syndrome is not clear. The vaginas of naturally infected hens are free of infection 1-3 mo after the source of infection is removed. Immunity is not permanent, and hens can be reinfected with contaminated semen.

Clinical Findings

Embryo infection appears to reduce hatchability, poult quality, and growth rate. Superimposed stress may cause considerable mortality in poults during the first few weeks. Infection during early rapid growth of hock joints, periarticular tissues, cervical vertebrae, and adjacent bone may produce major bone deformities such as crooked necks and hocks. Rales may develop in poults 3-8 wk old and persist for several weeks without significant mortality or serious interference with growth.

Lesions

Day-old poults have thoracic airsacculitis with thickening, turbidity, and marked caseous exudate. In 1-3 wk, the lesions may extend to the abdominal air sacs. These lesions recede with age. The air sac lesions of roaster and mature birds are probably related to other factors. Tracheitis may be present, but sinusitis does not occur.

Microscopic lesions in hens consist of lymphocytic foci in the fimbria, uterus, and vagina. In young poults, inflammatory lesions are seen in the air sacs and lungs.

Diagnosis

A high incidence of air sac lesions in day-old poults suggests M meleagridis infection. The serum plate agglutination or ELISA test may be used. Confirmation is generally by hemagglutination-inhibition, isolation and identification of the organism, or both. M gallisepticum, chlamydiae, bacteria, and respiratory viruses such as influenza must be eliminated as causes of air sac infection.

Treatment and Control

The commercial use of flocks free of M meleagridis should be monitored by serology and/or by examining pipped embryos or cull poults for airsacculitis. Semen used for insemination must be free of M meleagridis. Dipping eggs in tylosin or another suitable antibiotic reduces the incidence of transmission in infected flocks and may improve weight gains and feed conversion ratios. Inoculation SC of a suitable antibiotic at 1 day of age or water medication for the first 5-10 days appears to reduce airsacculitis caused by M meleagridis and may improve weight gain.

Mycoplasma Synoviae Infection

M synoviae was first recognised as an acute to chronic infection of chickens and turkeys that produced an exudative tendinitis and bursitis; it now occurs most frequently as a subclinical infection of the upper respiratory tract. M synoviae infection is also a complication of airsacculitis in association with Newcastle disease or infectious bronchitis. It is seen primarily in chickens and turkeys, but ducks, geese, guinea fowl, parrots, pheasants, and quail may also be susceptible. Serum (preferably swine serum) and nicotinamide adenine dinucleotide are required for growth on artificial media.

Transmission, Epidemiology, and Pathogenesis

M synoviae is egg-transmitted, but the rate is low (probably <5%), and some hatches of progeny may be free of infection. Egg transmission is greatest during the first 1-2 mo after infection of susceptible breeders. Lateral transmission is similar to that of M gallisepticum, but the rate of spread is generally more rapid.

M synoviae isolates vary widely in pathogenicity. Isolates from cases of airsacculitis are more apt to produce air sac lesions than isolates from synovial fluid or membranes. Some strains produce the typical clinical disease of synovitis. The paucity of natural outbreaks of clinical synovitis in chickens in recent years may be related to the adaptation of M synoviae to the respiratory tract; however, clinical synovitis in turkeys is relatively common.

Clinical Findings

Although slight rales may be present in birds with respiratory infection, usually no signs are noticed. Younger birds, especially those under stress or suffering concurrent infections, are more likely to be affected. Outbreaks of infectious synovitis occur most commonly in chickens at 4-6 wk and in turkeys at 10-12 wk. Lame birds tend to sit. The more severely affected birds are depressed and are found around the feeders and waterers. Swellings of the hocks and footpads are seen. Morbidity is 2-15%, and mortality 1-10%. The effect on egg production is minimal, but instances of egg production losses have occurred.

Lesions

In the respiratory syndrome, airsacculitis occurs when the bird is stressed from Newcastle disease, infectious bronchitis, or improper ventilation. In many cases, air sac lesions resolve after 1-2 wk. Early in synovitis, the liver is enlarged and sometimes green. The spleen is enlarged, and the kidneys are enlarged and pale. A yellow to gray, viscid exudate is present in almost all synovial structures; it is most commonly seen in the keel bursa, hock, and wing joints. In chronic cases, this exudate may become inspissated and orange.

Diagnosis

A presumptive diagnosis can be based on the lesions and clinical signs, but laboratory confirmation is necessary. Skeletal abnormalities must be eliminated as the cause of lameness. The disease must be differentiated from viral tenosynovitis and from staphylococcal and other bacterial infections.

The serum plate agglutination or ELISA test is used to detect infected flocks, but cross-reactions with M gallisepticum and other nonspecific reactions may occur. Reactors are confirmed as positive by hemagglutination-inhibition or by isolation and identification of the organism. PCR may be used to rapidly detect the organism in infected tissues. In turkeys, the agglutination test for M synoviae may not be reliable.

Treatment and Control

Serologic testing and isolation similar to those for M gallisepticum have resulted in eradication of the infection in most primary breeder flocks of chickens and turkeys. Administration of a tetracycline antibiotic in the feed may be beneficial in treatment or prevention of synovitis. When airsacculitis is a problem, preventive antibiotic therapy during the time of respiratory reaction to Newcastle disease and infectious bronchitis vaccine may be helpful. Medication of breeder flocks is of little value in preventing egg transmission.

Salmonelloses

Historically, the 3 salmonellae infections in poultry causing severe economic losses are Salmonella pullorum, S gallinarum, and S arizonae. Through the institution of control programs, the incidence of infections with these salmonellae has decreased dramatically. In addition to the above salmonellae, S paratyphoid infections in poultry are relatively common and have public health significance because of the consumption of contaminated poultry products. S pullorum and S gallinarum are highly host-adapted to chickens and turkeys. S arizonae is most important in turkeys, with chickens occasionally affected. There are ~2,000 nonhost-adapted species (paratyphoid) that may be transmitted to almost all animals.

Pullorum Disease

Etiology and Transmission

Infections with Salmonella pullorum usually cause very high mortality (potentially approaching 100%) in young chickens and turkeys. In adult chickens mortality may be high, but frequently there are no clinical signs. Pullorum disease was once common but has been eradicated from most commercial chicken stock, although it may occur in other avian species (eg, guinea fowl, quail, pheasants, sparrows, parrots, canaries, and bullfinches). Infection in mammals is rare. Transmission is primarily through the egg but also occurs via direct or indirect contact with infected birds. Infection transmitted via egg or hatchery contamination usually results in death during the first few days of life up to 2-3 wk of age.

Clinical Findings and Lesions

Affected birds huddle near a heat source, are anorectic, appear weak, and have whitish faecal pasting around the vent (diarrhea). Survivors frequently become asymptomatic carriers with localised infection of the ovary. Some of the eggs laid by such hens hatch and produce infected progeny. Lesions in young birds usually include unabsorbed yolk sacs and classic gray nodules in the liver, spleen, lungs, heart, gizzard, and intestine. Firm, cheesy material in the ceca (cecal cores) and raised plaques in the mucosa of the lower intestine are sometimes seen. Occasionally, synovitis is prominent. Adult carriers usually have no gross lesions but may have nodular pericarditis, fibrinous peritonitis, or hemorrhagic, atrophic regressing ovarian follicles with caseous contents. In mature chickens, chronic infections produce lesions that are indistinguishable from those of fowl typhoid.

Diagnosis

Lesions may be highly suggestive, but diagnosis should be confirmed by isolation, identification, and serotyping of S pullorum. Infections in mature birds can be identified by serologic tests, followed by necropsy evaluation complemented by microbiologic culture and typing for confirmation. Official testing recommendations are outlined in the USA National Poultry Improvement Program (NPIP).

Treatment and Control

Treatment of infected flocks to alleviate the perpetuation of the carrier state is not recommended. Control is based on routine serologic testing of breeding stock to assure freedom from infection.

Fowl Typhoid

Etiology and Epidemiology

The causal agent is Salmonella gallinarum. The incidence of fowl typhoid is low in the USA and Canada, but much higher in other countries. Although S gallinarum is egg-transmitted and produces lesions in chicks and poults similar to those produced by S pullorum, there is a much greater tendency to spread among growing or mature flocks. Mortality in young birds is similar to S pullorum infection but may be higher in older birds.

Clinical Findings and Lesions

Clinical signs and lesions in young birds are similar to those of infection with S pullorum. The older bird may be pale, dehydrated, and have diarrhea. Lesions in the older bird may include a swollen, friable, and often bile-stained liver, with or without necrotic foci, enlarged spleen and kidneys, anaemia, and enteritis.

Diagnosis

Diagnosis should be confirmed by isolation and identification and serotyping of S gallinarum (NPIP testing procedure).

Treatment and Control

Treatment and control are as for pullorum disease. There are no federally licensed vaccines in the USA. In other countries, vaccines (killed or modified live) made from a rough strain of S gallinarum (9R) have been useful in controlling mortality.

More recently, vaccines derived from outer membrane proteins, mutant strains, and a virulence-plasmid-cured derivative of S gallinarum have shown promise in protecting birds against challenge. The standard serologic tests for pullorum disease are equally effective in detecting fowl typhoid.

Arizona Infection

Etiology, Clinical Findings, and Lesions

Many serotypes have been identified from various birds, mammals, and reptiles. Foodborne infections occasionally occur in humans. Reptiles, wild birds, rats, and mice are frequently infected and are thought to act as a reservoir of infection for poultry.

Clinical signs and lesions are not distinctive. Mortality is usually limited to the first 3-4 wk of age, and adult carriers may not develop appreciable clinical signs. Infection tends to persist in a flock. Poults are diarrheic, listless, and unthrifty; in some flocks, birds may develop eye opacity and blindness. Neurologic signs occur due to infection of the brain.

Lesions include unabsorbed yolk sacs, enlarged and mottled livers, congestion in the duodenum, and caseous cecal cores. Some birds develop peritonitis, salpingitis, local ovarian infections, or ophthalmitis. Purulent material may be seen in the meninges.

Diagnosis

Diagnosis is based on isolation and identification of the organism. Affected eyes and brain are excellent sites for isolation. Environmental samples also may be used for detecting the microbe. Egg transmission levels are often high; therefore, culture of dead embryos, eggshells, and cull poults may identify infected breeding stock. Effective serologic tests have not been developed.

Treatment and Control

Killed vaccines (bacterins) have been used in infected breeder flocks to reduce egg transmission and to develop breeding flocks free of S arizonae. Early fumigation of hatching eggs and rigorous hatchery sanitation also aid in reducing transmission. Antibiotics are given by injection to day-old poults to minimise mortality. Birds may still carry and shed the organism even after treatment.

Paratyphoid Infections

Etiology, Clinical Findings, and Lesions

Paratyphoid infections can be caused by any one of the many nonhost-adapted salmonellae. These *Salmonella* may infect many types of birds, mammals, reptiles, and insects. Paratyphoid infections are of public health significance via contamination and mishandling of poultry products. Salmonella typhimurium, S enteritidis, and S heidelberg are among the most common salmonella infections in poultry, although infections may be produced by 10-20 different serotypes in the USA. Some species or strains are more pathogenic than others. The prevalence of other species varies widely by geographic location and season.

Transmission usually occurs horizontally from infected birds, contaminated environments, or infected rodents. With the exception of S enteritidis, transmission of most serotypes to progeny from infected breeders is mainly through faecal contamination of the eggshell. Infected birds remain carriers.

Clinical Findings and Lesions

Although not common, clinical signs are sometimes seen in young birds. Mortality is most often limited to the first few weeks of age. Depression, poor growth, weakness, diarrhea, and dehydration are hallmarks of the disease, although these clinical signs are not distinctive. Lesions may include an enlarged liver with focal necrosis, unabsorbed yolk sac, enteritis with necrotic lesions in the mucosa, and cecal cores. Infections occasionally localise in the eye or synovial tissues. Conversely, there may be no lesions due to acute death caused by septicemia. Isolation, identification, and serotyping of the causal agent are essential for diagnosis. Serology is not highly reliable.

Treatment and Control

General control measures for the paratyphoid Salmonella include strict sanitation in the hatchery, fumigation of hatching eggs, pelleting of feed to destroy salmonellae, cleaning and disinfection of poultry houses, rodent control, and use of competitive exclusion products. Several antibacterial agents help prevent mortality but cannot eliminate flock infection. Maintenance of poultry in confinement and exclusion of all pets, wild birds, and rodents help prevent introduction of infection.

Salmonella enteritidis (a paratyphoid Salmonella serotype) is a major food safety concern, primarily for the egg-laying industry. Possible sources in commercial layers include transmission from breeders, contaminated environments, infected rodents, and contaminated feed. Transmission to progeny from breeders is mainly through eggshell contamination, although, unlike other paratyphoid

Salmonella, transovarial transmission may also occur. The NPIP now includes S enteritidis control measures in breeders, including depopulation of infected flocks, cleaning and disinfection of pullet and layer houses, extensive and improved rodent control programs, use of competitive exclusion products, vaccination, and proper handling and refrigeration of eggs.

Tuberculosis

Tuberculosis is a slowly spreading, chronic, granulomatous bacterial infection, characterised by gradual weight loss. All birds appear to be susceptible, although to variable degrees; pheasants seem to be highly susceptible, while the disease is uncommon in turkeys. Tuberculosis is more prevalent in captive than in wild birds. Tuberculosis is unlikely to occur in commercial poultry due to the short life span and husbandry practices used.

Etiology and Epidemiology

Mycobacterium avium *var avium* is the cause. Serologic identification of isolates is essential to differentiate strains of M avium that cause disease in chickens and birds (serovars 1, 2, and 3) from other serovars that fail to produce disease in these species. M tuberculosis has infrequently been isolated from parrots and canaries. M avium is very resistant; it can survive in soil for up to 4 yr, in 3% hydrochloric acid for e"2 hr, and in 4% sodium hydroxide for e"30 min. Tuberculosis is found worldwide, most commonly in small, barnyard flocks and in zoo aviaries; it is rarely found in young flocks. Wild birds, such as cranes, sparrows, starlings, and raptors, have been found to be infected. Tuberculosis has been found in emus and other ratites.

Infected birds with advanced lesions excrete the organism in their feces. Cadavers and offal may infect predators and cannibalistic flockmates. Rabbits, pigs, and mink are readily infected. Cattle exposed to contaminated feces may respond to mammalian tuberculin and to johnin. M avium may cause disease in humans; serovar 1, often isolated from tuberculous chickens, has been isolated from people with acquired immunodeficiency syndrome.

Clinical Findings and Diagnosis

Signs usually do not develop until late in the infection when birds become thin and sluggish, and lameness may be seen. In chickens, granulomatous nodules of varying size are usually found in the liver, spleen, bone marrow, and intestine. Some exotic species may have lesions in the liver and spleen without intestinal involvement, but bone marrow and small mesenteric nodules may be found. Lesions are not calcified.

Live birds may be tested with avian tuberculins, although these are of little value in birds that do not have wattles. Large numbers of acid-fast bacteria in smears from lesions provide a tentative diagnosis.

Control

Chemotherapy is ineffective. In commercial poultry flocks, relatively rapid turnover of populations, together with improved general sanitation, has largely eliminated this once common infection. Infected poultry should be destroyed, and housing facilities thoroughly cleaned and disinfected using cresylic compounds. Dirt-floored houses should have several inches of the floor removed and replaced with dirt from a place where poultry have not been maintained. All openings should be screened against wild birds. Avian tuberculosis in zoos is difficult to eradicate. New additions to the aviary should be quarantined for 2-3 mo. The movement of ratites through sales and the long life of these animals have made tuberculosis a major concern for ratite producers. Isolation of ratites purchased at sales is essential to prevent the introduction of tuberculosis into established flocks.

Infectious Bronchitis

Infectious bronchitis is an acute, rapidly spreading, viral disease of chickens characterised by respiratory signs, decreased egg production, and poor egg quality. Some strains of the causative virus, infectious bronchitis virus (IBV), are nephropathogenic. The latter strains produce interstitial nephritis resulting in significant mortality. Infectious bronchitis is of major economic importance to commercial chicken producers worldwide.

Etiology and Epidemiology

IBV, a coronavirus, is worldwide in distribution and has numerous serotypes. Two or more serotypes may be seen simultaneously in one geographic region. IBV is shed by infected chickens in respiratory discharges and feces. The highly contagious virus is spread by airborne droplets, ingestion of contaminated feed and water, and contaminated equipment and clothng of caretakers. Naturally infected chickens and those vaccinated with live IBV may intermittently shed virus for many weeks or even months. Virus infection in layers and breeders occurs cyclically as immunity declines or on exposure to different serotypes.

Clinical Findings

Signs occur after an incubation period of 18-48 hr. Spread to other birds is rapid, and morbidity may be nearly 100%. The nature and severity of the disease are influenced by the age and immune status of the flock and virulence of the causal strain. Young chickens cough, sneeze, and have tracheal rales for 10-14 days. Wet eyes and dyspnea may be seen, and facial swelling may also occur ccasionally, particularly with concurrent bacterial infection of the sinuses. In broiler chickens, IBV infection is a major cause of poor feed conversion, reduced growth rate, and condemnation of meat at processing. Nephropathogenic strains can produce interstitial nephritis with high mortality (up to 60%) in young chickens. In most outbreaks, however, mortality is 5%, although secondary bacterial infections may cause higher losses.

In layers, egg production may drop 5-50%, and eggs are often misshapen, thin-shelled, and contain watery albumen. Egg production and egg quality generally return to near normal levels in most birds on recovery.

Lesions

Respiratory tract lesions include mucoid exudate in the trachea and bronchi, generally without hemorrhage. Caseous plugs may be found in the trachea of young birds. Air sacs are thickened and opaque. Secondary bacterial infections in meat-type birds, especially with coliform bacteria, produce caseous airsacculitis, perihepatitis, and pericarditis. Nephropathogenic strains produce swollen, pale kidneys, with tubules and ureters distended with urates. In layers, urolithiasis is associated with virus infection and certain dietary factors.

Diagnosis

Diagnosis cannot be based solely on clinical signs because of similarities to mild respiratory forms of Newcastle disease, laryngotracheitis, and infectious coryza. Seroconversion or a rise in IBV antibody titre shown by ELISA, hemagglutination inhibition, or virus neutralisation tests can be used for diagnosis given a history of respiratory disease or reduced egg production. A definitive diagnosis is generally based on virus isolation and identification. Virus can be isolated by inoculation of bacteria-free tissue homogenates of trachea, cecal tonsils, and kidneys into 9 to 11 day old chicken embryos. Several blind passages of the virus may be necessary for isolation of some field strains. The virus produces embryo stunting, curling, and urate deposits in the mesonephros, with variable mortality. Because the virus exhibits great antigenic variation, the serotype should be identified if possible. Serotypes are conventionally identified with the aid of known serotype-specific chicken antisera in the virus neutralisation test. However, the virus neutralisation test is expensive, time consuming, and not readily available; therefore, it is not commonly used. A limited number of serotype-specific monoclonal antibodies (MAb) have been developed for serotyping purposes. However, direct application of MAb-based immunohistochemical procedures for detection of viral antigen in infected chicken tissues is not considered dependable because of the low concentration of the antigen in the tissues. The MAb have been best used after the virus is propagated by passage in chicken embryos, in which case the virus can be detected in the cells associated with the chorioallantoic membranes by immunofluorescence or immunoperoxidase staining, or in the allantoic fluid by ELISA.

Analyses of the viral genome for the purpose of identifying the virus serotype are now commonly used. These methods are based on the application of reverse transcriptase PCR (RT-PCR), using-specific oligonucleotide primers, to produce DNA copies of IBV genes, usually of the S1 part of the spike glycoprotein gene. Subsequently, the RT-PCR product is subjected to restriction fragment length polymorphism (RFLP) or analysed by nucleotide sequencing. For RFLP, the RT-PCR product is digested with a set of specific restriction endonucleases, and the digested nucleic acid fragments are separated by gel electrophoresis. The specific pattern of their separation in the gel is compared with those of the standard strains for identification.

Control

No available medication alters the course of the disease, although antibiotic therapy may reduce mortality due to secondary infections. Increasing the temperature in the poultry house and under the hover by 5-10°F (3-5°C) may lower mortality.

Attenuated vaccines used for immunisation may produce mild respiratory signs. Live vaccines are initially given to chicks 1-14 days old by spray, drinking water, or eyedrop. Revaccination is common. Live or adjuvanted killed vaccines are sometimes used in breeders and layers to prevent egg production losses.

Many serotypes are recognised, and a number of new or variant serotypes have been reported, which pose problems in immunisation and diagnosis. If possible, selection of vaccine should be based on knowledge of the prevalent serotype(s) on the premises. The most commonly used live vaccines in the USA contain strains of IBV serotypes Massachusetts, Connecticut, and Arkansas. Vaccination with selected variant serotypes is practised in some areas. Outbreaks with mortality due to nephritis have been associated with several variant strains in Australia and the USA. Infection with standard as well as variant serotypes have been associated with egg production losses in vaccinated layer flocks.

Miscellaneous Conditions of Poultry

Ascites Syndrome

Ascites is an accumulation of noninflammatory transudate in one or more of the peritoneal cavities or potential spaces. The fluid, which accumulates most frequently in the 2 ventral hepatic, peritoneal, or pericardial spaces, may contain yellow protein clots. Ascites may result from increased vascular hydraulic pressure, vascular damage, increased tissue oncotic pressure, decreased vascular oncotic (usually colloidal) pressure, or blockage of lymph drainage.

The most common cause of ascites is increased vascular hydraulic pressure in the venous system, which is most commonly caused by right ventricular failure (RVF) or hepatic fibrosis.

In poultry, RVF is usually secondary to valvular insufficiency and may result from inflammatory (myocarditis, valvular endocarditis) or degenerative disease of the myocardium or valves or from congenital heart disease. In turkeys, spontaneous cardiomyopathy (*Round Heart Disease of Turkeys: Introduction*) is a common cause of ascites. However, the most common cause of ascites in meat-type chickens is RVF in response to increased pulmonary arterial resistance. Pulmonary hypertension occurs frequently in chickens secondary to the hypoxia of altitude with resultant polycythemia and increased blood viscosity.

It also occurs frequently secondary to the red blood cell rigidity of sodium toxicity and less frequently from lung pathology. When ascites occurs at low altitudes in meat-type chickens, which have a high metabolic oxygen requirement, it is usually caused by primary or spontaneous pulmonary hypertension because of insufficient capacity of the pulmonary capillaries.

In poultry, liver damage may be caused by aflatoxin or by toxins from plants such as Crotalaria. In broiler chickens, obstructive cholangiohepatitis (caused by Clostridium perfringens infection) is the most common cause of the liver damage, which results in ascites. In both meat-type ducks and breeders, amyloidosis of the liver frequently causes ascites.

Pathogenesis and Epidemiology

Pulmonary hypertension syndrome (PHS) is caused by increased pressure in the pulmonary arteries when the heart tries to pump more blood through the lungs to meet the body's oxygen requirement. The resultant volume and pressure overload on the right ventricle cause dilatation and hypertrophy of the right ventricular wall, valvular insufficiency, RVF, and ascites.

Bird lungs are rigid and fixed in the thoracic cavity. The capillaries can expand very little to accommodate increased blood flow. Lung size in proportion to body weight, and particularly to muscle mass, decreases as meat-type chickens grow. Increased blood flow results in primary pulmonary hypertension and cor pulmonale with sporadic cases of RVF and ascites in fast-growing broilers.

Predisposing factors that increase oxygen demand (e.g., cold), reduce oxygen-carrying capacity of the blood (e.g., acidosis, carbon monoxide), increase blood volume (e.g., sodium), or interfere with blood flow through the lung (e.g., lung pathology that narrows or occludes capillaries, increased RBC rigidity, or polycythemia with increased blood viscosity) may result in flock outbreaks of PHS with or without ascites.

The incidence of PHS is >2% in some broiler and many roaster flocks and is occasionally 15-20% in other roaster flocks. Right ventricular hypertrophy is the response to an increased workload and eventually leads to RVF if the volume or pressure load persists. Hypertrophy of the right ventricular wall is directly related to pulmonary hypertension, and the ratio of the right ventricle to the total ventricular mass can be used as a measure of the increased pressure load on the right ventricle.

Clinical Findings

Occasionally, young broilers develop PHS, particularly if increased sodium or lung pathology (e.g., aspergillosis) is involved, but in primary pulmonary hypertension, mortality is greatest after 5 wk of age. Clinical signs are not seen until RVF occurs and ascites develops. Clinically affected broilers are cyanotic, the abdominal skin may be red, and peripheral vessels congested. Because growth stops as RVF develops, affected broilers may be smaller than their pen mates. However, rapid growth rate is a known predisposing factor, and sometimes the largest broilers are affected, with occurrence in males more frequent than in females. The ascites increases the respiratory rate and reduces exercise tolerance. Affected broilers frequently die on their backs, and differential diagnosis includes flip-over disease (*Flip-over Disease: Introduction*). Not all broilers that die from PHS have ascites. Death may occur suddenly before clinical signs are seen.

Lesions

Most lesions are the result of increased venous hydraulic pressure secondary to RVF. There is a variable amount of clear yellow fluid and clots of fibrin in the hepatoperitoneal spaces. The liver may be swollen and congested, or firm and irregular with edema, and have clotted protein adherent to the surface. It may be nodular or shrunken; it may be white with subcapsular edema and a thickened capsule, or have large or small blebs of fluid between the capsule and the visceral peritoneum. Hydropericardium is mild to marked, and occasionally there is pericarditis with adhesions. Right ventricular dilatation and mild to marked hypertrophy of the right ventricular wall may be noted. The right atrium and vena cava are very dilated. Occasionally, there is thinning of the left ventricle. The lungs are extremely congested and edematous. The intestine may or may not be empty.

Diagnosis

Broilers that die from ascites or suddenly as the result of RVF or pulmonary hypertension can be identified by the enlarged heart; enlarged, thickened right ventricle; or fluid in the body cavities and heart sac. If the wall of the right ventricle is enlarged or thickened, the broiler has probably died from PHS, even if there is no fluid in the body or heart sac.

Control

Reducing the birds' metabolic oxygen requirement by slowing growth or reducing feed can prevent ascites caused by PHS. Environmental temperature, humidity, and air movement should be controlled to prevent excessive loss of body heat, particularly in the early neonatal period. Ascites caused by other factors (e.g. sodium, lung damage, liver damage, etc.) can be prevented by avoiding the etiologic agents involved. Altitudes >3,000 ft (900 m) are unsatisfactory for meat-type chickens, and growth must be slowed to prevent mortality. More care to prevent chilling is also necessary at higher altitudes.

Breast Blisters

In chickens and turkeys, a bursa lined with synovial membrane normally exists over the anterior projection of the keel bone. When this bursa becomes inflamed by trauma or infection, fluid or exudate accumulates and appears as a fluid-filled blister 1-3 cm in diametre. Causes of trauma to this bursa include poor feathering, hard flooring, and leg weakness, which is associated with increased recumbency. Some young turkeys have pointed keels, which can lead to increased bursal trauma, but as the size of their breast muscle increases and trauma decreases, lesions may regress. Infectious causes of sternal bursitis include Mycoplasma synoviae, Staphylococcus, and Pasteurella spp.

Breast Buttons

These are lesions found in a similar location to breast blisters. They have a hard crust on the surface and a core of dead skin and granulomatous reaction extending into the subadjacent subcutis. Their etiology is not well defined but they are not due to the causes listed above for breast blisters. Rather they may be chemical burns due to prolonged contact of poorly feathered skin with wet litter containing ammonia or toxins.

Cannibalism

Cannibalism is an abnormal behaviour of chickens and turkeys most often manifested as vent-picking or picking at unfeathered skin on the head, comb, wattles, or toes. No single cause has been identified, but overcrowding, excessive light intensity, and nutritional imbalances are directly correlated with its occurrence. Additionally, in overly fat pullets entering egg production or hens in production, mucosa will protrude from the vent during and after egg laying, and this red tissue will attract pecking. Other factors that predispose to cannibalism are insufficient feeder space, mineral and vitamin deficiencies, skin injuries, and failure to remove dead birds daily. Other than the loss of birds due to pecking trauma, cannibalism often leads to transmission of infectious diseases (e.g. erysipelas) and botulism.

Control depends on correcting or reducing the above risk factors and trimming the sharp distal end of the upper beak to prevent pecking. Trimming of the tip of the beak distal to the nostrils is often done at 1 day of age and repeated between 6 and 12 wk of age in maturing pullets or turkeys. Cautery often is required to provide hemostasis.

Fluke Infections

Modern poultry production methods have diminished the incidence of fluke infections, although the parasites persist in poultry allowed contact with snails or other hosts and in some wild birds.

Prosthogonimus macrorchis, the oviduct fluke of poultry, infects birds after they consume infective metacercariae in larval or mature dragonflies, the secondary host. The fluke matures in ~2 wk in the bursa of Fabricius or, in gallinaceous birds without a functional bursa (e.g., chickens, turkeys, pheasants), in the oviduct.

Light infections without clinical signs appear in ducks and other birds with a functional bursa. In gallinaceous birds, heavy infections in the oviduct cause inappetence, droopiness, weight loss, calcareous cloacal discharge, depressed egg production, and an increase in soft-shelled eggs. Lesions range from mild inflammation to distention or rupture of the oviduct; death may result. Diagnosis by faecal examination is unreliable because fluke eggs are not consistently present. Adult flukes may appear in the bird's eggs or be found in the oviduct on necropsy.

To prevent fluke transmission, birds must be kept from feeding on dragonflies. There is no effective treatment approved for use in poultry. Carbon tetrachloride, a common remedy, is highly toxic to chickens and other birds.

Collyriclum faba, another common fluke in birds, appear as subcutaneous cysts 4-6 mm in diametre (usually containing 2 adults) anywhere on the body but more frequently near the vent in turkeys, chickens, and other birds. The cysts ooze an exudate, which attracts flies and predisposes to bacterial infection. Signs in young birds include locomotor difficulty and inappetence; death may result in heavy infections. The parasites can be removed surgically. The life cycle is unknown but probably involves snails and insects such as dragonflies or mayflies. Prevention of infection requires restricting birds from areas frequented by aquatic insects.

Gout

Avian species excrete nitrogenous wastes as urates bound in colloidal form with mucus in their urine. Renal disease decreases the clearance of uric acid from the blood, which results in acute or chronic hyperuricemia, and the excess uric acid precipitates on either visceral or articular surfaces (gout). Urate deposits are white and semisolid and must be differentiated from yellow fibrinous or purulent inflammatory exudates that are secondary to infectious causes such as synovitis, peritonitis, perihepatitis, and pericarditis.

Acute urate deposition occurs after rapidly progressing renal failure, or as a terminal event with acute decompensation of chronic renal disease. Deposits develop most commonly on the pericardium, peritoneum, and liver capsule, and rarely on synovial surfaces of joints and tendons. They are usually present for too short a time to induce significant inflammation. Most clinical cases of acute renal failure and urate deposition in commercial poultry are due to dehydration, ingestion of feed containing >3% calcium by nonlaying chickens, renal infection by nephrotropic strains of infectious bronchitis virus, or infection with avian nephritis virus. Other avian species commonly develop visceral deposits secondary to nephrotoxin exposure, most commonly aminoglycoside antibiotics or heavy metals.

Chronic urate deposition is less common and occurs after longterm increases in serum levels of uric acid. Deposits develop on synovial membranes in the toes and wing joints and incite a chronic granulomatous reaction to urate crystals (tophi). Chronic urate deposition may be seen in chickens that have hereditary defects in uric acid metabolism or that are fed excessive protein.

Urolithiasis is common in older laying chickens. Brittle, white, staghorn calcium urate calculi form in one or both ureters. Most cases are due to feeding high-calcium laying feed to hens not in egg production, infection with infectious bronchitis virus, or severe vitamin A deficiency. If blockage is complete, acute postrenal failure develops, and birds die with acute urate deposition on visceral surfaces or less commonly in joint spaces. If blockage is incomplete or unilateral, chickens survive in compensated renal failure, and chronic urate deposits form in joint spaces.

Pendulous Crop

Incidence of pendulous crop is low in flocks of chickens and turkeys. The crop is visibly distended and contains foul-smelling fluid, feed, and litter. Digestion is impaired, and affected birds become thin or emaciated. If these birds survive, they often are condemned or trimmed at processing to reduce contamination by ingesta.

The etiology is not known, but a hereditary predisposition has been suggested in turkeys. Incidence may increase with erratic feed or water consumption. Experimentally feeding rations containing cerelose as a substitute for starch can cause pendulous crops. Vagus nerve damage has also been postulated as a cause. There is no known efficacious treatment.

Colibacillosis

Colisepticemia, Escherichia Coli Infection

Colibacillosis occurs as an acute fatal septicemia or subacute pericarditis and airsacculitis. It is a common systemic disease of economic importance in poultry and is seen worldwide.

Etiology and Pathogenesis

Escherichia coli is a gram-negative, rod-shaped bacterium normally found in the intestines of poultry and most other animals; although most are nonpathogenic, a limited number produce extraintestinal infections. Pathogenic strains are commonly of the O1, O2, and O78 serotypes, but serotypes O11, O15, O18, O51, O115, and O132 have also been reported for E coli isolates associated with cellulitis and colibacillosis. There is considerable diversity of serogroups among clinical isolates, and only a small percentage of these isolates belong to serotypes O1, O2, or O78.

In fact, 18-29% of avian E coli isolates cannot be typed. Therefore, no single E coli serotype used as a bacterin can provide full protection against all of the serotypes that cause E coli infections. Virulence factors include the ability to resist phagocytosis, utilisation of highly efficient iron acquisition systems, resistance to killing by serum, production of colicins, and adherence to respiratory epithelium. Virulent E coli are generally nontoxigenic, poorly invasive, and do not possess common adhesins.

Large numbers of E coli are maintained in the poultry house environment through faecal contamination. Initial exposure to pathogenic E coli may occur in the hatchery from infected or contaminated eggs, but systemic infection usually requires predisposing environmental factors or infectious causes. Mycoplasmosis, infectious bronchitis, Newcastle disease, hemorrhagic enteritis, and turkey bordetellosis precede colibacillosis. Poor air quality and other environmental stresses may also predispose to E coli infections.

Systemic infection occurs when large numbers of pathogenic E coli gain access to the bloodstream from the respiratory tract or intestine. Bacteremia progresses to septicemia and death, or the infection extends to serosal surfaces, pericardium, joints, and other organs.

Clinical Findings and Lesions

Signs are nonspecific and vary with age, organs involved, and concurrent disease. Young birds dying of acute septicemia have few lesions except for enlarged, hyperemic liver and spleen with increased fluid in body cavities. Birds that survive septicemia develop subacute fibrinopurulent airsacculitis, pericarditis, perihepatitis, and lymphocytic depletion of the bursa and thymus. (Unusually pathogenic salmonellae produce similar lesions in chicks.) Although airsacculitis is a classic lesion of colibacillosis, whether it results from primary respiratory exposure or from extension of serositis is unclear. Sporadic lesions include pneumonia, arthritis, osteomyelitis, and salpingitis.

Diagnosis

Unlike pathogenic E coli associated with illnesses in other animal species, avian isolates are generally nonhemolytic on sheep (5%) blood agar. Isolation of a pure culture of E coli from heart blood, liver, or typical visceral lesions in a fresh carcass indicates primary or secondary colibacillosis. Consideration should be given to predisposing infections and environmental factors. Pathogenicity of isolates is established when parenteral inoculation of young chicks or poults results in fatal septicemia or typical lesions within 3 days. Pathogenicity can also be detected by inoculation of the allantoic sac of 12 day old chick embryos. Resulting gross lesions include cranial and skin hemorrhages in addition to encephalomalacia in embryos inoculated with virulent isolates.

Treatment and Control

Treatment strategies include attempts to control predisposing infections or environmental factors and early use of antibacterials indicated by susceptibility tests. Most isolates are resistant to tetracyclines, streptomycin, and sulfa drugs, although therapeutic success can sometimes be achieved with tetracycline. In fact, 90% of clinical isolates are resistant to tetracycline, with 60% of isolates resistant to 5 or more antibiotics. Fluoroquinolone use is controversial because the use of these drugs in commercial broilers is believed to select for resistant Campylobacter spp associated with human foodborne infections. Commercial bacterins, administered to breeder hens or chicks, have provided some protection against homologous E coli serotypes.

Duck Viral Hepatitis

Duck viral hepatitis is an acute, highly contagious, viral disease of young ducklings characterised by a short incubation period, sudden onset, high mortality, and characteristic liver lesions. The disease is of economic importance in all duck-raising areas of the world. Three distinct types of duck hepatitis virus (DHV) have been isolated from diseased ducklings. A natural outbreak of DHV Type I has been reported in mallard ducklings; experimental DHV Type I infections have been produced in goslings, turkey poults, young pheasants, quail, and guinea fowl. The viruses that cause hepatitis in ducklings should not be confused with duck hepatitis B virus, a hepadnavirus infection of older ducks.

Etiology

The originally described, most widespread, and most virulent DHV Type I is an enterovirus in the family Picornaviridae and is readily propagated in chick and duck embryos. It does not produce hemagglutinins. Field experience with DHV Type I indicates that egg transmission does not occur. The disease can be transmitted experimentally by parenteral or oral administration of infected tissues.

Viruses differing from classic DHV Type I have been recognised as causes of hepatitis in ducklings. DHV Type II is considered to be an astrovirus and is difficult to propagate under laboratory conditions;

DHV Type III is a member of the Picornaviridae, is antigenically distinct from Type I virus, and can be propagated in duck (but not chick) embryos. A distinct serologic variant of DHV Type I, named DHV Type Ia, has also been described.

Clinical Findings

The incubation period for Type I virus is 18-48 hr. Affected ducklings become lethargic, lose balance, paddle spasmodically, and die within minutes, typically with opisthotonos. Although adults may become infected, clinical signs have not been seen in ducks >7 wk old. Mortality may be as high as 95% in ducklings. Practically all deaths occur within 1 wk after onset of signs. The clinical course of DHV Type II infection is similar to that of Type I and can occur in ducklings immune to Type I infection. DHV Type III infections occur in ducklings despite immunity to Type I virus. The clinical course of Type III infection is less severe, and mortality is rarely >30%.

Lesions

The lesions caused by all 3 types of DHV are similar. The liver is enlarged and covered with hemorrhagic foci up to 1 cm in diametre. The spleen may be enlarged and mottled. Kidneys may be swollen, and renal blood vessels congested.

Diagnosis

A presumptive diagnosis can be based on the history and lesions. Sudden onset, rapid spread, and short course, together with characteristic liver lesions, are highly suggestive of duck viral hepatitis. Type I virus may be isolated in duck embryos, day-old ducklings, and duck-embryo liver cell cultures, or less easily in chicken embryos. The virus can be identified by neutralisation with specific antisera or by inoculation into both susceptible and immune ducklings. Type II and III viruses are not neutralised by classic Type I antiserum.

Prevention and Treatment

Prevention is by strict isolation, particularly during the first 5 wk of age. Contact with wild waterfowl should be avoided. Rats have been reported as a reservoir host of the virus; therefore, pest control is indicated.

Immunisation of breeder ducks with modified live virus vaccines, using Type I, II, and III viruses, provides parenteral immunity that effectively prevents high losses in young ducklings. The Type I virus vaccine is administered SC in the neck to breeder ducks at 16, 20, and 24 wk of age and every 12 wk thereafter throughout the laying period. Three immunisations are advisable for passive protection of ducklings.

An inactivated DHV Type I vaccine for use in breeder ducks that have been previously primed with live DHV Type I virus has been described. A single dose of the inactivated vaccine, given IM before the birds come into lay, provides passive immunity for a complete laying cycle to progeny ducklings.

The chick-embryo origin, modified live Type I virus vaccine also can be used for early vaccination of ducklings susceptible to Type I (progeny of nonimmune breeders). This vaccine is administered SC or by foot web stab in a single dose to day-old ducklings. Vaccinated ducklings rapidly develop an active immunity over 3-4 days.

Antibody against Type I virus, prepared from the eggs of hyperimmunised chickens, administered SC in the neck at the time of initial loss, is an effective flock treatment.

Enterococcosis

The application of new bacteriologic techniques, especially DNA-DNA and DNA-rRNA hybridisation has led to the reclassification of Lancefield group D streptococci as Enterococcus spp. (For a discussion of diseases caused by the Lancefield antigenic serogroup C and other Streptococci spp).

Enterococcus spp in avian species are worldwide in distribution. Enterococci are ubiquitous in nature and commonly found in various poultry environments. Enterococcus spp are considered normal microflora of the intestinal tract of poultry and other birds. A high percentage of ready-to-eat poultry products are contaminated with Enterococcus spp; however, no resultant food poisoning in humans has been reported.

Etiology and Epidemiology

The genus Enterococcus is composed of gram-positive, spherical bacteria occurring singly, in pairs, or in short chains, which are nonmotile, non- sporeforming, facultative anaerobes. They are catalase-negative and ferment sugars, usually to lactic acid. Common avian isolates can be differentiated by their ability to ferment mannitol, sorbitol, and L-arabinose and by their growth on MacConkey agar without crystal violet or salt. (Other types of MacConkey agar inhibit Enterococcus and may provide false-negative results.) Enterococcus spp isolated from avian species and associated with disease include E faecalis, E faecium, E durans, E avium, and E hirae. E faecalis affects birds of all ages; it is a serious disease occurring in embryos and young chicks from faecal-contaminated eggs. E faecium is a cause of mortality in ducklings.

Enterococci are transmitted most commonly via oral and aerosol routes. However, transmission can occur through skin injuries, especially in caged layers. Aerosol transmission of E faecalis results in acute septicemia in chickens. Concurrent enteric infections or any condition compromising the intestinal villous epithelium, allowing penetration of resident enterococci, can result in septicemia, bacterial endocarditis, or both. Incubation periods range from 1 day to several weeks, with 5-21 days most common. Endocarditis can occur when a septicemic enterococcal infection progresses to a subacute or chronic stage. Enterococcus spp have been associated with brain necrosis and encephalomalacia in young chickens. Some enterococci, however, have been demonstrated to have a beneficial effect on growth and feed efficiency and are being studied as potential probiotics.

Clinical Findings

Enterococcus spp in poultry can result in 2 distinct clinical forms of disease, acute and subacute/chronic. In the acute form, clinical signs are related to septicemia and include depression, lethargy, lassitude, pale combs and wattles, ruffled feathers, diarrhea, fine head tremors, and decrease or cessation of egg production. Often, only dead birds are found. In the subacute/chronic form, depression, loss of body weight, lameness, and head tremors may be observed. Body temperature is elevated in birds with persistent bacteremia. Clinically affected birds eventually die if not treated. Egg transmission or faecal contamination of hatching eggs results in late embryo mortality and an increased number of chicks or poults unable to "pip" or penetrate through the shell at hatch.

Lesions

Gross lesions of enterococci infection in acute disease include splenomegaly, hepatomegaly (with or without foci), enlarged kidneys, and congestion of subcutaneous tissue. Omphalitis or enlarged yolk sacs may be seen in chicks or poults infected at hatching. Hepatomegaly, splenic necrosis, fibrinous pericarditis, perihepatitis, and airsacculitis are observed in ducks infected with E faecium. Lesions of chronic enterococcal infections include fibrinous arthritis and/or tenosynovitis, osteomyelitis, fibrinous pericarditis and perihepatitis, necrotic myocarditis, and valvular vegetative endocarditis similar to that observed with Streptococcus zooepidemicus infection. Additional gross lesions associated with valvular endocarditis include an enlarged, pale, flaccid heart; pale to hemorrhagic areas in the myocardium; infarcts in the liver, spleen, or heart; and, less commonly, infarcts in the lung, kidney, and brain.

On microscopic examination, the liver has dilated sinusoids congested with RBC and increased heterophils. Splenomegaly is characterised by congestion and hyperplasia of cells in the mononuclear phagocytic system. Valvular lesions consist primarily of fibrin with bacteria, heterophils, macrophages, and fibroblasts. Other microscopic lesions related to endocarditis include cerebral vasculitis and infarcts, leptomeningitis, glomerulonephritis, and thrombosed pulmonary vessels. Focal granulomas can be found in virtually any tissue as a result of septic emboli. Aggregates of bacteria are present throughout necrotic areas with a zone of heterophils just within the necrotic border, a characteristic feature of the lesion. Gram-positive bacterial colonies are readily observed in thrombosed vessels and within necrotic foci.

Diagnosis

Demonstration of bacteria typical of enterococci in blood or impression smears of affected heart valves or lesions from birds with typical clinical signs will provide a presumptive diagnosis of enterococcosis. Isolation of Enterococcus spp (without faecal contamination) from typical lesions will confirm the diagnosis. Enterococci are easily isolated on blood agar or more specific differential media, which should help differentiate species. Fermentation of mannitol, sorbitol, and arabinose, and growth on MacConkey agar (without crystal violet or salt) can also aid in differentiating enterococci from Streptococcus spp. Preferred tissues for culture include liver, spleen, blood, yolk, embryo fluids, or any suspected lesion. Diagnosis of bacterial endocarditis is based on valvular vegetations with secondary infarcts of myocardium, liver, or spleen. In suspected cases, it is important to culture lesions to establish a definitive diagnosis and rule out other bacteria.

Differential diagnosis includes other bacterial septicemic diseases, e.g., staphylococcosis, streptococcosis, colibacillosis, pasteurellosis, and erysipelas.

Treatment and Prevention

Treatment includes use of antibiotics such as penicillin, erythromycin, novobiocin, oxytetracycline, chlortetracycline, or tetracycline in acute and subacute infections. Clinically affected birds respond well early in the course of the disease. As the disease progresses within a flock, treatment efficacy decreases. Antibacterial sensitivity should be performed on bacterial isolates in any clinical cases of enterococcosis before treatment begins. There is no treatment for poultry with bacterial endocarditis.

Prevention and control requires reducing stress and preventing immunosuppressive diseases and conditions. Proper cleaning and disinfection can reduce environmental enterococcal resident flora to minimise external exposure.

Erysipelas

Erysipelas in poultry is seen worldwide, mainly as an acute septicemia. Outbreaks usually occur suddenly, with a few birds being found dead followed by increasing mortality on subsequent days. Mortality may range from <1% to 50%. From an economic standpoint, turkeys are the most important poultry species affected, but serious outbreaks have occurred in chickens, ducks, and geese. Mammals are also affected, with swine being the most economically important species. Infection in reptiles and amphibians has also been reported. The organism has been isolated from the surface slime on fish, which may serve as a source of infection for other species. People usually become infected when the organism enters through cuts in the skin. There have been no reports of people becoming infected by the oral route. The disease in humans (erysipeloid) is most common in people who handle infected tissues such as veterinarians, butchers, and fish handlers. Erysipeloid in people may be a localised or a septicemic and occasionally fatal infection.

Etiology

The causative agent is Erysipelothrix rhusiopathiae, a facultatively anaerobic, intracellular bacterium. A second genomic species, E tonsillarum, has been described but is not considered pathogenic for poultry. Morphologically, E tonsillarum cannot be distinguished from E rhusiopathiae. E rhusiopathiae stains gram-positive but tends to decolourise, particularly in older cultures. The organism is nonmotile, does not form spores, and produces no known toxins. There is no flagellum but a capsule has been demonstrated. The cellular morphology of E rhusiopathiae is variable. Cells freshly isolated from tissues during acute infection or from smooth colonies are straight or slightly curved small rods that may occur in short chains. Cells from older cultures or rough colonies tend to become filamentous and may be confused with mycelia. The filamentous form occurs more frequently after repeated passages on artificial media.

E rhusiopathiae grows readily on ordinary culture media containing the blood or sera of various animals. Growth is enhanced by reducing the oxygen content or increasing the carbon dioxide level to 5-10%. Optimal incubation temperature is 35-37°C, and the optimal pH range is 7.4-7.8.

The organism is not readily destroyed by the usual laboratory disinfectants, and it may survive in litter or soil for various lengths of time; therefore, disinfection of premises is difficult. E rhusiopathiae may also survive smoking and pickling processes. It is inactivated by a 1:1,000 concentration of bichloride of mercury, 0.5% sodium hydroxide solution, 3.5% liquid cresol, 5% solution of phenol, or 0.5% formalin.

Though different serotypes of E rhusiopathiae exist, no correlation has been shown to exist between the serotype, chemical structure, or biochemical pattern, and the manifestation of the septicemic, urticarial, or endocardial forms of erysipelas.

Epidemiology

Erysipelas occurs sporadically in poultry of all ages. Turkeys are susceptible regardless of sex or age. Recent evidence indicates that there may be a genetically related resistance in turkeys. The incidence in males is reported to be higher, but this is not supported by experimental data. Erysipelas may affect the fertility of males and may contribute to downgrading and processing losses. Infection results from entrance of the organisms through breaks in the skin, through the mucous membranes such as during artificial insemination, by ingestion of contaminated foodstuffs (particularly cannibalism of infected carcasses), and possibly by mechanical transmission via biting insects. Fighting and cannibalism increase losses.

The organism is shed in feces from infected animals and contaminates the soil, in which it may survive for long periods depending on temperature and pH. Seasonal changes in climate such as the onset of cold, rainy weather have been associated with disease occurence. Poultry, as well as other animals, may be carriers and shed the organism without showing clinical signs of disease.

In nonvaccinated flocks, morbidity and mortality may reach 40-50%, but mortality is usually limited to <15%. In vaccinated flocks, some birds may be depressed for a short period and recover. Mortality in vaccinated and nonvaccinated poultry is influenced by the virulence of the organism.

Clinical Findings

Erysipelas is primarily an acute infection that results in sudden death. In an affected flock, a few birds may be depressed but easily aroused; within 24 hr, a few birds will be dead. Just before death, some birds may be very droopy, with an unsteady gait. Chronic clinical disease in a flock is not usual but does occur; birds may have cutaneous lesions and swollen hocks. Turkeys with vegetative endocarditis usually do not have clinical signs and may die suddenly. Erysipelas should be suspected in flocks that have been artificially inseminated 4-5 days before an episode of death without clinical signs. Clinical signs in chickens include general weakness, depression, diarrhea, and sudden death. In laying hens, egg production may drop markedly.

Lesions

At necropsy, a generalised darkening of the skin or various sized areas of diffuse darkening is common. The liver and spleen are usually enlarged and friable and may be mottled. There may be other gross lesions such as peritonitis, pericarditis, catarrhal exudate in the GI tract, and degeneration of fat associated with the thigh and heart.

Bibliography

Abbas, M.A.: *Effect of Organic Amendments and EM on Crop Production in Pakistan,* SP, Brazil. Pub. USDA. Washington, D.C., 19991.

Ahn., D.U. : *Effects of Post-Mortem Time Before Chilling and Chilling Temperatures on Water Holding Capacity and Texture of Turkey Breast Muscle,* Poultry Science, 1997.

Andrew L. Winton: *Poultry Eggs,* Agrobios, Delhi, 2002.

Ball, W.: *Egg Quality Guidelines for the Australian Egg Industry,* AECL Publication, UK, 2004.

Bhosale, Dinesh T. : *Handbook of Poultry Nutrition,* International Book, 2004.

Bourke, M.: *Beak Trimming Handbook for Egg Producers,* Landlinks, UK, 2006.

Chandra, Rajesh : *Diseases of Poultry and Their Control,* IBDCO, Delhi, 2001.

Charles, T. Burr and Homer O. Stuart: *Commercial Poultry Farming,* Biotech Books, Delhi, 2011.

Chenoweth, H.: *Free-Range Poultry,* Free-Range Poultry Production and Marketing, Creola, Ohio, 2001.

Cotterill, O.J.: *Egg Science and Technology,* Food Products Press, Imprint of Haworth Press, New York, London, 1995.

Cox, N. A. : *Relationship Between Aerobic Bacteria, Salmonella, And Campylobacter on Broiler Carcasses,* Journal of Food Protection, 1997.

Cramer, C.: *Sustainable Farming Connection: Where Farmers Find and Share Information,* Sustainable Farm Publishing, US, 1997.

Dennis Wages: *Biosecurity in the Poultry Industry,* International Book, Delhi, 2006.

Elson, H.A.: *Poultry Production Systems, Behaviour, Management and Welfare,* CAB International, NY, 1992.

Fanatico, A.: *Pastured Poultry: A Heifer Project International Case Study Booklet,* Little Rock, AR, 2000.

Ferguson, M.W.J.: *Egg Incubation, Its Effects on Embryonic Development in Birds and Reptiles,* Cambridge University Press, UK, 1991.

Foreman, P.: *The Chicken Tractor: The Permaculture Guide to Happy Hens and Healthy Soil-All New Straw Bale Edition,* Good Earth Publications, USA, 2002.

Fraser, AF & Broom, DM.: *Farm Animal Behaviour and Welfare,* CABI, UK, 2004.

Fries., R. : *Air Chilling and Evaporation Technique in Poultry Meat Production- A Microbiological Survey II. Differentiation,* Fleishwirtschart,1997.

Garnsworthy, P.C.: *Recent Developments in Poultry Nutrition,* University Press, India, 1999.

Gillespie, J.R.: *Modern Livestock and Poultry Production 7th edition,* Thomson Delmar Learning, 2004.

Grist, A.: *Poultry Inspection, Anatomy, Physiology and Disease Conditions,* Nottingham University Press, UK, 2006.

Hambidge, Gove : *Diseases and Parasites of Poultry,* Biotech Books, Delhi, 2004.

Hatta, H.: *Hen Eggs: Basic and Applied Science,* CRC Press, Delhi, 1996.

Haunshi, Santosh : *Objective Poultry Science,* Daya Pub, Delhi, 2011.

Hernandez, J.: *Optimum Egg Quality: A Practical Approach,* 5M Publishing, U.K, 2007.

Hill, Donna *: Biosecurity in the Poultry Industry,* International Book, 2006.

Hunton, P.: *Poultry Production,* Elsevier, 2007.

Hurd, Louis M : *Modern Poultry Farming,* Greenworld, Delhi, 2003.

Jull, Morley A. : *Successful Poultry Management,* Biotech, Delhi, 2001.

Keith Wilson N.D.P: *A Handbook of Poultry Practice,* Agrobios, Delhi, 2000.

Lakhotia, R.L. : *Agro's Dictionary of Poultry Science,* Agrobios, Delhi, 2006.

Leclercq, B.: *Nutrition and Feeding of Poultry,* Nottingham University Press, U.K., 1994.

Leeson, S & Summers, J.D.: *Scott's Nutrition of the Chicken,* University Books, UK, 2001.

Leeson, S. and J.D. Summers: *Commercial Poultry Nutrition,* Nottingham University Press, Delhi, 2008.

Mandal, A.B. : *Nutrition and Disease Management of Poultry,* International Book Distributing Co, Delhi, 2004.

McLelland, J.: *A Colour Atlas of Avian Anatomy,* Wolfe Publishing, London, 1990.

Mead, G.: *Food Safety Control in the Poultry Industry,* Woodhead Publishing Limited, Abington Hall, Abington, Cambridge, 2006.

Mead, G: *Poultry Meat Processing and Quality,* CRC Press, USA, 2004.

Moguilevsky, M. A. : *Drug Resistance of Enterobacteriacaea Isolated from Chicken Carcasses,* Journal of Food Protection, 1997.

Mohiuddin, S M : *Moulds and Mycotoxins in Poultry Diseases,* International Book, Delhi, 2007.

Mudd, D.: *Profitable Poultry: Raising Birds on Pasture*, USDA's Sustainable Agriculture Network (SAN), Washington, DC, 2001.

Nandi, S. and S. Samanta: *Poultry Diseases: At a Glance*, IBDC Pub, Delhi, 2010.

Nicholls, C.: *The Workboot Series: The Story of Eggs in Australia*, Kondinin Group, Cloverdale W.A., 2005.

North, M.O.: *Commercial Chicken Meat and Egg Production*, Kluwer, USA, 2001.

Nowland, W.J.: *Modern Poultry Management in Australia*, Rigby, 1978.

Owen, W Powell : *Poultry Farming and Keeping*, Biotech Books, Delhi, 2005.

Panda, A K ; S V Rama Rao and M R Reddy: *Growth Promoters in Poultry : Novel Concepts*, International Book Dist, Delhi, 2008.

Pathak, N.N. *: Nutrition and Disease Management of Poultry*, International Book Distributing Co, Delhi, 2004.

Perry, G.: *Welfare of the Laying Hen*, CABI Publishing, UK, 2004.

Powell., C. : *Microbiological and Hydraulic Evaluation of Immersion Chilling for Poultry*, Journal of Food Protection, 1995.

Prasad, L N *: Advanced Pathology and Treatment of Diseases of Poultry : With Special Reference to Etiology Signs*, International Book Dist, Delhi, 2006.

Prasad, Sushil : *Handbook Of Poultry Production : A Practical Guide*, Enkay Publishing House, Delhi, 2011.

Rai, Manoj Kumar : *Handbook Of Poultry*, Oxford Book Company, Delhi, 2011.

Randall, C.J.: *Color Atlas of Diseases and Disorders of the Domestic Fowl and Turkey*, Iowa State University Press, UK, 1991.

Randall, V . : *Mutagenicity of Poultry Chiller Water Treated With Either Chlorine Dioxide or Chlorine*, Journal of Agricultural and Food Chemistry, 1997.

Reddy, M R *: Growth Promoters in Poultry : Novel Concepts*, International Book Dist, Delhi, 2008.

Reddy, V. Ramasubba and Dinesh T. Bhosale: *Handbook of Poultry Nutrition*, International Book, Delhi, 2004.

Renema, R.A.: *New Developments in Reproduction and Incubation of Broiler Chickens*, Spotted Cow Press, Ltd, Edmonton, Alberta, Canada, 2003.

Roberts,V.: *Diseases of Free-Range Poultry: Including Hens, Ducks, Geese, Turkeys, Pheasants, Guinea Fowl, Quail and Wild Waterfowl*, Whittet, UK, 2000.

Ru, Y.: *Developing Free-Range Animal Production Systems*, RIRDC, US, 2004.

Sainsbury, D.: *Poultry Health and Management*, Blackwell Science, US, 2000.

Saxena, H.C. : *Poultry Feed Technology : Feed Formulation and Manufacturing*, International Book, Delhi, 2006.

Schade, R.: *Bioactive Egg Compounds,* Springer, Delhi, 2007.

Sharma, R.P. : *Poultry Production in India*, Indian Council of Agricultural Research, Delhi, 2007.

Sharma, RN : *Poultry Management*, Vista International Publishing House, Delhi, 2008.

Sharma, S.R. *: Poultry Production in India*, Indian Council of Agricultural Research, 2008.

Shukla, Rakesh Kumar *: Handbook of Poultry Diseases : A Bedside-Guide*, International Book Dist, Delhi, 2006.

Singh, C D N ; S D Singh; S P Verma and L N Prasad: *Advanced Pathology and Treatment of Diseases of Poultry : With Special Reference to Etiology Signs*, International Book Dist, Delhi, 2006.

Singh, Ram Prakash : *Modern Livestock and Poultry Production*, Biotech Books, Delhi, 2008.

Sreenivasaiah, P V *: Scientific Poultry Production : A Unique Encyclopaedia*, International Book Dist, Delhi, 2006.

Stephen F. Strausberg: *From Hills and Hollers: Rise of the Poultry Industry in Arkansas,* Arkansas Agricultural Experiment Station, Fayetteville, 1995.

Steven, K .L. : *Potent Bacterial Mutagens Produced by Chlorination of Simulated Poultry Chiller Water*, Journal of Agricultural and Food Chemistry, 1996.

Swan. S E J *: Small-Scale Poultry Production : Technical Guide*, Daya, 2007.

Thyagarajan, D. : *Diseases of Poultry*, Satish Serial pub, Delhi, 2011.

Tsushima, T. : *Survey of Bacterial Contimanation and Microbiological Control at a Poultry Slaughterhouse*. Journal of the Japan Veterinary Medical Association, 1996

Vegad, J L *: Poultry Diseases : A Guide for Farmers and Poultry Professionals*, International Book Dist, Delhi, 2008.

Verma, S. S. : *Microbiological Changes on Chicken Carcasses During Processing*, Indian Journal of Poultry Science, 1989.

Watson, R.: *Eggs and Health Promotion,* Iowa State Press, UK, 2002.

Whitehead, C.C.: *Bone Biology and Skeletal Disorders in Poultry*, Carfax Publishing Company, U.K., 1992.

Wilson, G.C.: *Egg Quality Handbook,* NSW DPI, MT, 1990.

Young, M.: *Controlling Newcastle Disease in Village Chickens*, ACIAR, US, 2002.

Index

□□□